"In Peggy Horan's inspired hands, Esalen massage becomes a true practice in the spiritual sense, based on intimate connections between people. Read this book for both the "how" and the deeper "why" behind the techniques, and experience the wonder for yourself."
—GORDON WHEELER, PH.D., president and CEO of the Esalen Institute and author of *Beyond Individualism: A New Perspective on Self, Relationship, and Experience*

"Touch is its own, unique form of communication, which can foster genuine understanding between partners in ways that words alone cannot. For more than thirty years, I have been dazzled by Peggy Horan's extraordinary talents and sensitivities. She is truly one of the great living masters of the art of massage. In *Connecting Through Touch*, she does a superb job of capturing all of the ways in which touch can comfort, stimulate, bridge gaps, and heal. I have every confidence that this book will enrich the relationships of anyone who reads it."
—KEN DYCHTWALD, PH.D., author of *Bodymind, The Age Wave*, and *The Power Years*

"Don't miss this sophisticated, accurate, delightful approach to bodywork."
—JACK LEE ROSENBERG, DDS, PH.D., founder and director of Integrative Body Psycho therapy in Venice, CA

"For many in the Esalen Community, touch was the first door to self-discovery. In this book, Peggy Horan leads us into the wonderful world of touch. You couldn't find a better guide."
—CHRISTINE PRICE, teacher at and long-time resident of the Esalen Institute

"Some aspects of a relationship lie deeper than words. Peggy Horan rolls together our human needs for pleasure, communication, and well-being in this practical guide for couples massage. Couples can strengthen their partnerships as well as get rid of those achy back pains by giving each other massages with these principles in mind. Our divorce rate could plummet!"
—BRITA ORSTROM, LMFT, a founder of the Esalen Massage School and family therapist with a background in somatic, body-based psychotherapy

CONNECTING THROUGH TOUCH

the couples' massage book

PEGGY MORRISON HORAN

New Harbinger Publications, Inc.

Distributed in Canada by Raincoast Books

Copyright © 2007 by Peggy Morrison Horan
New Harbinger Publications, Inc.
5674 Shattuck Avenue
Oakland, CA 94609
www.newharbinger.com

Cover and text design by Amy Shoup and Sara Christian;
Large cover image by George Doyle/Stockbyte/Getty Images;
Other cover images by Brock Bradford; Interior images by Brock Bradford
Acquired by Jess O'Brien; Edited by Jess Beebe

Library of Congress Cataloging-in-Publication Data

Horan, Peggy Morrison.
  Connecting through touch : the couples' massage book / Peggy Morrison Horan.
    p. cm.
  ISBN-13: 978-1-57224-502-0 (pbk. : alk. paper)
  ISBN-10: 1-57224-502-6 (pbk. : alk. paper)
  1. Massage. 2. Couples. I. Title.
RA780.5.H67 2007
615.8'22--dc22
                    2007044741

09 08 07

10 9 8 7 6 5 4 3 2 1   First printing

DEDICATION

This book is dedicated to my husband, Richard: my life partner, my first masseur, and the one who still gives me the best backrub in the world.

CONTENTS

ACKNOWLEDGMENTS

My biggest thanks go to Esalen Institute for its dedication to making a better world, one human heart at a time. My thanks for being there and gently cradling me as I grew and learned and developed in ways I never imagined. My appreciation goes to all of my inspired teachers and fellow practitioners at Esalen, where we have been blessed to work together for almost four decades at the sacred waters where the art of Esalen massage was created.

In addition, I thank the good people at New Harbinger: Jess O'Brien, Jess Beebe, and Amy Shoup, as well as the many others whom I never met but who contributed time and energy to this project.

And finally, my thanks to my daughters: Jasmine, for your tireless editing of my early ramblings, and Lucia and partner Carsten Hunter, for being my beautiful models.

FOREWORD

My first massage, in my early twenties, was memorable in that I had no idea how to simply lie back and receive it. It was truly overwhelming to feel my body melting into a pair of strange hands. Thoughts like *Shouldn't I say or do something or get up right now and pull myself together* were floating through my head. As hard as I resisted surrendering, I finally fell all the way down to the bottom of myself, and nothing had ever felt so good.

I'm not sure I would be sitting here today without the ten thousand massages that I have experienced since then. They have moved me through the highs and lows that organically come with life: the losses, the celebrations, the disappointments, and the stresses, as well as the ordinary plateaus of contentment or boredom. Massage has been my vehicle of resurrection and renewal. It has helped me to see the dreams trapped in my thighs, to feel the breaths held hostage in my belly, to sense the memories etched into the soles of my feet. And all I have to do is stay present and follow the hands, like guides, through the wilderness of my body, back to my most essential self.

And I am still learning to let go (to this day, my right arm resists giving in to another's will), to relax, to feel the ecstatic bliss of being an embodied spirit. For Westerners, this is a lifelong mission. Many of us have been totally disconnected from the cathedral of our own bones and banished from the inner sanctum of our own body, often unwittingly by those whom we love. Reclaiming the body is as political a statement as it is personal. As we do this, we are also reclaiming the power and beauty of our sweet planet Earth. One does not exist without the other.

It has been my blessing to be on the receiving end of many massages with my dear friend and colleague, Peggy Horan. Every practitioner has a style. In my experience, Peggy is the queen of flow, one stroke blending seamlessly into the next, creating a continuous roll of rhythm calling me to take refuge deep within myself. Over the years, her dedication to her practice has exposed her to techniques from all over the world. She has integrated much body wisdom into her hands, into her heart, and now, through her words, into our hands and hearts.

Peggy's book represents the next leg on our journey. Now is the time to integrate massage into our homes, into our bedrooms, and into our relationships with our loved ones. I remember a fifteen-year-old boy who participated in my massage workshop because he wanted to learn how to massage his grandmother's aching feet. Recently, a cabdriver in Manhattan hit a bicyclist across the street from a medical conference I was attending. A massage practitioner grabbed her essential oils and ran out to give whatever she could to both freaked-out men. One of the cops who arrived on the scene said, "Wow, come with us, we need you!" Sometimes massaging a shoulder or a neck speaks louder than all the words we can muster, to say, *You are not alone here.*

For me, massage is a spiritual practice for both giver and receiver. In everything is the seed of its apparent opposite, and in no practice is this more apparent than in the ordinary act of reaching out to touch another. We need each other. We each possess the power to heal, and this power can only move through creative action. We, who have been so lost, desperately need keys to unlock the wisdom of affection and intimacy in safe, natural, and organic ways. Massage is such a tool. And this poetic yet practical book is such a guide.

—Gabrielle Roth,
October, 2007

INTRODUCTION

Being touched and caressed, being massaged is food for the infant. Food as necessary as minerals, vitamins, and proteins. Deprived of this food, the name of which is love, babies would rather die. And they often do. —Frederick Leboyer, *Loving Hands*

My first massage was given to me by my husband. He was not my husband at the time. He was a handsome young artist who had come to Big Sur hoping to pursue his art and live a life closer to the land. He was making his living giving massages at Esalen Institute. I was a young New Yorker, exploring the cutting edge of the culture at Esalen, a center for the exploration of human potential. I had never experienced massage until my first visit there.

Esalen is located on the magical California coast, where the mountains dramatically meet the sea. The hot sulfur springs that gush from the cliffs offer their healing waters to bathers, as they have since the days of the original caretakers of the land, the Esselen Native Americans. The beauty of the place, combined with the openness of those who lived there, completely enchanted me. Esalen was exploring cultural changes, pushing the boundaries of the known, and the times were ripe with questioning institutions and beliefs regarding life, love, psychology, religion, and spirituality.

I moved to Big Sur in the fall of 1969, unsure of what I would do there, knowing only that it was a place of truth for me and I had a lot to learn. For a while I worked in the Esalen kitchen as a dessert cook, and I soon found this was not my path. I was very drawn to massage. I loved receiving a session on the deck of the baths, warmed by the sun, feeling the oil penetrate my thirsty skin and sore muscles, feeling the tenderness and presence of my practitioner. I was moved in new ways and was beginning to feel what I was looking for, which was a deeper connection to my soul, a sense of balance in my own body, mind, and spirit. I felt compelled to learn this art, this craft, this healing practice that felt so deep and so profound. I began to study Esalen massage.

DISCOVERING ESALEN MASSAGE

My teachers were those who helped develop the practice in the 1960s: Storm, Seymour Carter, Bernie Guenther, Gabrielle Roth, Richard Horan, Robert DeLong Miller, and Vicki Topp. There were many others, including all the loving practitioners I have worked with over my long career at Esalen. Each practitioner brings his or her own special gift to the work, so the more teachers I worked with, the more textured my work became. Some taught me presence, some grace, some technique, and some how to open my heart.

Esalen massage was an emerging art. The form, which was originally based on Swedish massage, began to change as the teachers' ideas and influences were blended into the technique and each practitioner brought his or her particular expression to the work.

Freedom, in all its forms, was what many were seeking. Celebration of life, expression of feelings, and being in the here and now was guiding much of the study at Esalen at that time. Eastern mysticism was beginning to blend with Western thought. There was a huge spiritual awakening and cultural change beginning at Esalen, and Esalen massage evolved from this culture of the sixties.

Of particular interest to me was the study of the human body. The connection between body, mind, and spirit was being recognized and science was beginning to take seriously the notion of the mind affecting tissue and vice versa. The thinking was changing to bodymind, instead of body and mind. Our bodies hold our memories, and life experience is stored in our cells. Even unconscious thought is expressed in our bodies, in the way we hold tension and the way we move. As these ideas were becoming more accepted, psychologists began looking at the body for answers.

Massage and bodywork evolved along with changes in thinking as cutting-edge teachers flocked to this mecca of exploration of consciousness. Esalen massage continues to evolve and change to this day, incorporating movement and forms from many other disciplines and styles and cultures.

The discovery I made in my first massage class was such a joyful surprise: I experienced giving of myself to be the true gift. This language without words was one I could speak from my heart. It felt both comfortable and natural to me. Massage met my need to make people feel good. I loved the sensual feeling of skin on skin, the rhythmic slow pace, and the care and tenderness with which the client was approached.

I also loved the concept that the client and I were working together, that an exchange of energy was taking place. We were communicating and connecting through this language of touch, a language that came from a very deep place in me, one that perhaps I knew instinctively yet had forgotten. I loved that I could give tenderness in this beautiful way and that touch alone could awaken such deep feelings. I was so moved the first time I massaged a client and he cried because he had never been touched in such a loving way before!

There was so much room for creativity, for intuition, and for healing through this loving work. Some people are not given their birthright of the love from their family, the security of a loving caress, or the emotional nourishment needed to grow and flourish. For some, touch is associated with pain or fear. It was clear to me that through the nurturing and skill of the practitioner's sensitive touch, massage could help begin to heal those wounds of deprivation.

I began to discover in myself my own body/mind and spiritual connection. I was exploring and opening my senses, my mind, and my heart in so many new ways. There was a broad offering of study at Esalen. There were massage and sensory awareness classes, where we were guided through exercises designed to awaken all of our senses and show us how to become present in the moment. There was yoga and tai chi, where we explored breathing and balance and movement. There was gestalt awareness practice and exploration of group dynamics through psychodrama and encounter. We practiced meditation, learning focus and presence. All of these practices influenced me, both by nurturing my ability to be present and by awakening my senses and heightening my awareness. My sensitivity developed as I began to incorporate what I'd learned into my practice of massage.

It soon became clear that this work was healing not only for the recipient, but also for me. I loved the meditative, quiet place I would go to give a massage. I loved that the work itself was a moving meditation, like a dance with pulses and rhythms that emerged effortlessly and allowed me to move gracefully. I loved how I could be intuitive and compassionate with clients, that I could infuse my practice with yoga principles and enjoy the physical workout, without putting stress on my own body. I loved the sighs and the breaths and the smiles and the tears and hugs of thanks from grateful clients who experienced touch in a way that felt sacred. I loved that the work was received on deeps levels, way beneath the skin, closer to the soul, where clients experience their sense of real self, their feelings, and their emotional home inside their body.

HOW COUPLE MASSAGE BEGAN FOR ME

Since the very beginning of our relationship, my husband and I have always traded massages. He was a potter in those days, spending many hours hunched over a potter's wheel moving wet clay into form. At the end of the day, his back was tired from potting and from tending our garden and his many farm animals, as was mine from massaging clients, lifting children, and doing chores. We were living at Esalen in our early days together, in a tree house, a literal one with no bath. We used the Esalen hot tubs regularly. The hot sulfur water helped to relax our tired muscles, and we often traded massages—sometimes in the sun, sometimes at sunset, or in the evening, when it was very quiet and peaceful at the baths.

As life got busier for us, we had less time to do the full exchange and began to do "spot work" on each other, focusing on the areas of tension. Generally, it was my husband's back that troubled him. His shoulders were tight; his mid back needed stretching, weight, and pressure. His muscles were crying to be firmly kneaded. I loved having my shoulder muscles squeezed and my back massaged. My lower back always welcomed counterpressure and stretching.

We found ways to work with each other simply by trying different techniques. We always gave each other feedback, and over the years, we have come to know each other's bodies and problem areas, and we've learned how to work with each other. We have gotten a lot more specific in our work, and even if we have only a few minutes, we take the time for a quick massage, and it always makes a big difference in the way we feel.

The other benefit is the time we spend together, sharing and making each other feel good, listening to each other, and being present for each other. This is nourishment for any partnership, and it has helped sustain us through rough times as well as good times.

This began over thirty-five years ago for me, and the work became not only my job, but my practice, a way of developing mindfulness, a meditation. My husband and I continue to work on each other, and over time we have developed some of our own methods, which I will share with you in the following chapters.

WHAT THIS BOOK OFFERS

The book begins with preparation for the massage and then addresses giving and receiving a basic full-body massage using a massage table. I've also included creative ways to work with each other when there is no table. A massage doesn't have to be an hourlong treatment. There are so many ways to share this work that fit into your life easily and naturally.

Although much of the book is dedicated to the craft of massage, I also address the art, and ways to develop that art. By the art, I mean the way to connect with yourself, so your mind is quiet and you can hear your intuitive senses and your creativity can emerge. Learning technique gives you a framework and the tools to practice massage; the art of the work will emerge. As your focus on the technique fades, you will become more confident and more able to move from a place of feeling, rather than from thought. The craft can be learned, and the art is from the heart.

I encourage couples to use this book as a guide to learning the fundamentals of massage and to develop your own ways of working together. It is useful to read it through once and then return to it as you practice, using it as a guide. Feedback—including asking for what you want—is an important element in making this work enjoyable for you. Communication must be clear and honest.

The book is meant to inspire you and give you some tools to develop the practice of massage, and in the process, to develop compassion for each other, to nourish your relationship, and to deepen your connection. Relationships must be fed. Couples don't live happily ever after without putting some time and energy into making that happen. Sharing massage becomes a loving way to communicate, to speak through the language of touch instead of words. Loving attention is expressed through your presence and sensitive touch.

We live in a culture where it is becoming accepted that touch heals. We see spas and healing centers in many towns, and bodywork is offered almost everywhere, even in businesses and airports. Massage is becoming a household word, and hallelujah for that! How natural, then, it is to bring home and share this loving, healing art with your partner. Who could be more qualified to offer that to each other?

The first chapter of this book prepares the giver and receiver, and explains the importance of the basic principles of quality of touch and presence and listening. The following chapters include exercises in learning touch, as well as massage techniques that can be used with and without a massage table. Take what feels good to you and try it. Experiment, explore, and develop creative ways of massaging each other that feel right for you and your partner. Use this book as a guide but not a bible. There are many ways to work, and I encourage you to find your own style. My hope is that you will be inspired to share with your beloved, as well as family members and friends, the deep connection and healing that this practice offers and to make it a special part of your lives.

Ashley Montagu, in his groundbreaking work *Touching* (Harper and Row, 1981), describes the "mind of the skin" (4) and writes that the sense of touch is the earliest sense to develop. The embryo begins to respond to stimulation and stroking as early as six weeks, and continues to react to stimuli throughout gestation. Our skin receives the first touch at birth, and the stimulation and love given through that touch helps us to thrive. Even when we're adults, the need for touch is always there, and between couples, touch serves as glue that helps hold a relationship together. Sexual contact is one way for touch to find expression. It is possible to bring touch into your communication in many other ways: a gentle hand when someone's had a bad day, a stroke of the head in passing, a hug for no reason, a hand held in a scary movie or while crossing the street. By repressing touch, we close down our other senses and our ability to communicate wordlessly. When words are not enough, where else can we go? Massage is food for the relationship, nourishment for the body and soul, and a gift to share throughout your lives.

I'll teach you massage through words and pictures, but the feeling you put into it will come from your heart. Relax and be open to the exercises and suggestions that follow. I offer them to help awaken your senses and feelings, to open your heart to the love inside, and to show you how to touch each other deeply with it. Enjoy giving as much as receiving. Allow the intimacy to bathe you as you become more comfortable with this silent language of love.

CHAPTER 1

PREPARING FOR THE MASSAGE

Before beginning a massage, it is important to prepare your environment, externally as well as internally. In this chapter, I'll discuss practical aspects like massage oils and the massage table. I'll also offer exercises to help each of you quiet your mind, develop a sense of touch, and cultivate the kind of communication that enhances both giving and receiving.

PREPARING THE EXTERNAL SPACE

Massage is an inherently relaxing activity, and the massage environment can contribute to the experience.

The Massage Room

Create a personal sacred space that is both private and comfortable. Quiet is optimal, and warmth is essential. Some people like to massage outside in the sun or shade, while others prefer the intimacy of a fireside massage or the coziness of the bedroom. The space must be comfortable for both of you. When you are giving, you stay warmer because you are moving, so it is best to make the space warm enough for the receiver, who is still.

If you choose to work outside, make sure there is ample protection from the sun. Sunblock, as well as shade, prevents serious burning from lying in the sun with oil on your skin.

If you are indoors, unplug your telephone so the sound doesn't interrupt you. There is nothing worse than the phone ringing when you're deeply relaxed. Choose a room where there is no traffic, put on some soft music if you like, and if there are children in the house, make sure another adult is watching them so your time together is uninterrupted.

Use candles or soft lighting. Some couples like to create an altar in their massage space. The altar can be made of a collection of objects you consider special, such as stones, art, statuary, found objects, or photos. By approaching your surroundings in a ritualistic way, you create a special environment in which to work. Give yourselves the gift of time together in a space created especially for you, with none of life's interruptions.

The Massage Table

To give an entire massage to each other, it is best to have a massage table. You can purchase one easily online, or borrow one at first to try it out. If there is a massage school in your area, you can ask to see their tables and often pick up a used one from the school or one of their practitioners. Unless you have the space to leave the table set up all the time, I suggest an aluminum-legged table that can be folded and stored when not in use. They are light and can be moved around easily, especially if you purchase the outer cover, which has carrying straps to go over your shoulder for support. Extra padding under the vinyl makes the table more cushy and comfortable. Tables usually come with a detachable face cradle, which is used to support the head in the prone position. This prevents the receiver from getting a sore neck by lying with the head turned to one side. These tables are easily adjustable at the legs, making them suitable for givers of any height.

Cover the table with a soft sheet (a twin size will work). Flannel feels good, particularly in cool climates. Cover your face cradle so the receiver's skin doesn't touch the plastic. You can purchase a cover made especially for the face cradle, or you can use a folded pillowcase. You can use a sheet, towel, or sarong for draping, whichever is most comfortable for you both. There are bolsters made of foam and vinyl to support the ankles when the receiver is lying facedown. If you do not have a bolster, use a pillow at the foot of the table for ankle support. Place it under the sheet so it stays clean. This support helps take pressure off the lower back, and its height will depend on the comfort of the receiver. Some people prefer to let their ankles rest at the foot of the table with their feet off the end.

Massage Oil or Lotion

Oil or lotion is used to provide lubrication and allow moves that don't pull the skin. They make the contact feel smooth. The use of oil as opposed to lotion is matter of personal choice. Some people's skin works better with lotion, some with oil, depending on the dryness of the skin and how the lubricant is absorbed. Some people prefer the way one feels over the other. Both are cool to the skin when first applied, so it's a nice touch to warm the lotion or oil before applying it to the skin. You can put the plastic bottle in warm water for ten minutes to bring it to body temperature or slightly warmer.

Whether you use oil or lotion, find one with the least amount of preservatives in it, since the thirsty skin of the both the giver and the receiver absorbs the chemicals. If you're using oil, cold-pressed vegetable or nut oil (if you are not allergic to nuts) are best because the skin absorbs them well and they contain healthy nutrients. Organic products with no preservatives are best. Jojoba oil, apricot kernel oil, or sweet almond all make good massage oil and don't have their own strong odor. They should be kept in a cool place and used within a month or two, before they go rancid. You can always tell by the smell, so if your oil has been around for a while, give it the sniff test before using. There are many commercial massage oils and lotions now available. Read the labels to know what you are getting, or make your own by choosing a base lotion or oil and blending it with others and adding essential oils. If you have an allergy to nuts, use only the vegetable oils.

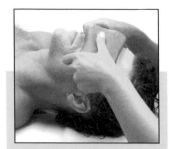

EYE PILLOWS

If you like, have an eye pillow handy for the faceup portion of the massage. An eye pillow is an herb-filled silk bag that covers the eyes, keeping the light out. It feels soft and comforting on the eyes and encourages an inward journey.

Essential oils

Essential oils are concentrated essences of plants, flowers, fruits, and herbs. They have been used throughout history as both perfume and medicine. The most effective way to use essential oils in massage is as a scent. Several drops added to your massage lotion can further your partner's ability to relax. Lulled by the lovely sensuous smell of the oil, your partner will soon be breathing more deeply.

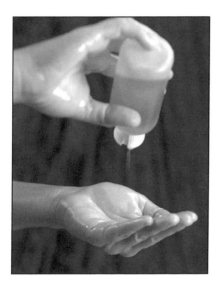

There are many essential oils to choose from. Offer your partner the bottle of essential oil to smell before adding it to the base oil or lotion. Women seem to enjoy the flower essences, such as jasmine, lavender, and rose, while men sometimes prefer the woody tones, such as sandalwood and cedar. Again, look for the purest oils available and don't use the synthetics. Three or four drops added to your base oil or lotion should be enough to scent it nicely. You can add more if you like it stronger. Not only do these essential oils help invite relaxation, they can have a therapeutic effect on the whole body and are used medicinally to support change, balance, and healing.

Personal Hygiene

There are a few things to remember regarding your personal hygiene. A shower or bath prior to the massage is always best for both the giver and receiver. That way you both start fresh and clean.

Giver, trim your fingernails so as not to scratch the receiver's skin. Clean your hands and fingernails, and make sure your breath is fresh. Keep your hair brushed back and remove any jewelry on your fingers or wrists. Wear comfortable clothes that allow you to move freely. Your shirt should fit well so as not to fall in your partner's eyes. Bare feet will allow you to move quietly about the table.

PREPARING THE INTERNAL SPACE

The practice of massage begins with the giver. By this I mean that the giver's energy is passed on in whatever form it exists. If you are distracted, anxious, angry, or otherwise not present, these are the qualities that come through your touch. Whatever you feel in the moment is what you pass on to your partner. A deeper connection is more possible if both partners are fully present and relaxed. A quiet mind and supportive, loving presence help you to feel compassion. This form of presence is what allows the receiver to feel safe and to begin to let go of the tension held in the cells. This sense of safety is particularly important for those who have a history of inappropriate touch or are not yet comfortable being massaged, even by their partner. It's important to honor each other by acknowledging the past as part of what influences the present. Take care not to reinjure your partner by an insensitive touch. Honest, open communication is essential to good massage.

A Quiet Mind

In this world of multitasking, moments of total presence can be rare. Total presence means being fully engaged in the moment, in body, mind, and spirit. Exercises and spiritual practices have developed over the centuries that use breath to connect body, mind, and spirit. (Yoga is one such practice.) These practices help you learn how to quiet the mind and how to be in the moment.

You may already have a meditation practice and find coming to a quiet state of mind easy and familiar. Or perhaps it is new, and it may take some time for you to feel comfortable doing this practice. I can't emphasize enough the importance of learning to quiet your mind before giving a massage. Not only will a quiet mind bring you into the moment, into your sense of self and what you're feeling, but it also creates the conditions for listening to your partner. Quiet presence is fertile ground for *intuition*, that sense of knowing without being told. Compassion, too, is developed with focus and attention. This is when the practice becomes art.

The following exercises are offered to give you some tools for becoming more fully present. They enable you to share what can become a deep practice.

sitting meditation

Let's start with a simple sitting practice. A sitting practice allows you to come into stillness by sitting and focusing on your breath. Gradually your mind begins to

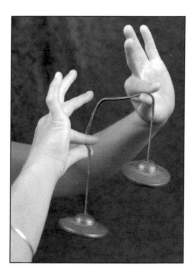

quiet as you let go of thoughts and just stay connected to your breath and your body. You will begin to feel present, with no thoughts and no agenda.

I suggest you wear comfortable clothing, with nothing binding at the waist, and take off your shoes and socks. Agree on how much time you want to spend in meditation together. If you are beginning this practice, limit your sitting time to whatever is comfortable. Maybe do three to five minutes the first time, then five, then ten or more. Decide which of you will track the time and close the meditation by softly sounding a small chime or bell.

1 Find a comfortable way to sit facing each other, but not touching. Use a meditation pillow on the floor, sit cross-legged, or use a chair with a straight back.

2 Sit with your spine straight and your hands resting comfortably on your lap, palms open. Take a moment to adjust your position so you feel balanced and feel the support of the floor or chair firmly beneath you. You should be balanced on the bones of your buttocks, with your spine comfortably straight, allowing the natural curves of your spine.

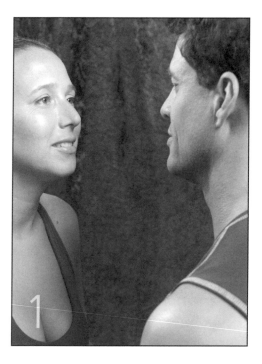

3 Now, take a deep breath and slowly exhale, allowing all the air to leave your lungs. Gently close your eyes. Follow your inhalation and exhalation through several deep breaths.

4 If you're holding tension in your body, observe it and know that it's natural. Try experiencing the expansion and contraction of every cell in your body in response to your breath. Notice how your ribs and your chest move in rhythm to maintain this balance of expansion and contraction, yin and yang. Honor this breath as the lifegiving gift it is and welcome the path it creates into your inner being. Continue to breathe consciously.

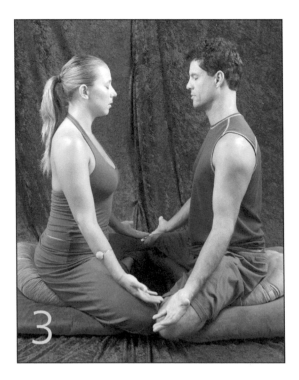

5 Bring your awareness to your chest and to your heart. Observe your feelings in the moment. Imagine your heart opening. Continue to follow your inhalation and your exhalation.

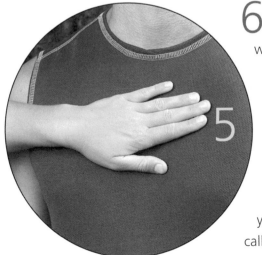

6 Now bring your breath and attention to your belly, just below your navel. Three fingerwidths below the navel is your center, or *hara*, as the Japanese call it. It is a place within you that is quiet, grounded, and calm. The seat of this refuge is deep in your belly. You can go here to feel grounded and comfortable in yourself and to connect in the deepest sense to your source of power. For many people, this is home. Let your breath fill your belly, and feel this home in yourself. Send your breath there, as you rhythmically inhale and exhale.

7 Notice how your mind wants to wander, and bring your attention back to your breath. Your mind is a trickster, constantly trying to tempt you away from your focus. When you find you've wondered off somewhere in your past or future, return to your breath and the present time. Your breath is always there to bring you back.

8 Observe how your breath begins to slow down after you've been sitting in stillness for a while. You may need to move or make some adjustments to your position to remain comfortable. Let your attention rest with your breath as you repeat this conscious inhalation and exhalation in your own time. After a while, you will notice that your mind begins to quiet.

9 After the agreed-on time has passed and the timekeeper has indicated the close of the meditation with a quiet sound, take your time and come back very gradually. After several breaths, and only when you feel ready, very slowly open your eyes, allowing the light to enter a little at a time. Maintain a soft gaze for a moment. Take in the room slowly, and finally let your eyes rest on each other. Allow the silence and breathe together. Enjoy this moment without the need to speak or to do anything. Continue to be in silence together as your prepare for the next exercise.

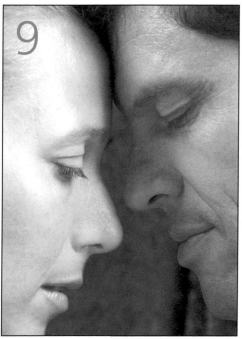

This sitting meditation offers you the opportunity to be quiet together in your busy lives. Like any other practice, this can grow with time and offer you the ability to find peace and stillness within yourself as well as the ability to ground and center yourself by using your breath. This is the place from which to begin a massage, with a quiet mind and a sense of connection.

Developing a Sensitive Touch

Learning to touch with sensitivity is central to learning massage. Technique means nothing without quality of touch. What makes a "good" touch, as opposed to a "bad" one? You would probably agree that you want the person touching you to be present, calm, and centered and the touch to be sensitive and firm yet gentle and nurturing. You want to feel safe and not invaded, and most of all, you want a loving touch, especially from your partner. Now, let's begin with an exercise in sensitivity practice.

sensitivity practice

If you have completed the meditation and are seated together, you can stay where you are for this exercise. Otherwise, come together in a seated position facing each other, close but not touching yet.

1 Take a moment to connect to yourself by taking some deep breaths. Notice your thoughts, notice where your attention goes, and bring your awareness back to your breath. As you sit together and your breathing slows down, let your breath fall into a pattern together and breathe as one for several minutes.

2 Bring your attention to your hands and turn your palms face up. Notice the sensations in your hands. You may feel warmth or cold, tingling or pulsing, or even anticipation in your fingertips.

3 Bring your palms slowly to your heart and hold them against your body as you take another deep breath. Notice any feelings in your chest as you do this. Feelings become more accessible to you when you bring your awareness to the fullness of your breath in your chest and abdomen.

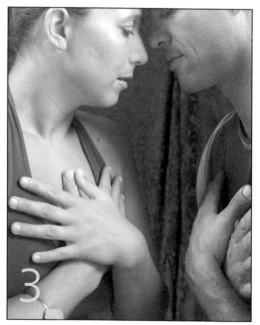

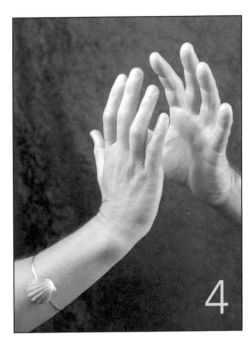

4 Now turn your palms to face your partner and again notice the sensations in your hands.

5 Now begin to bring your palms closer together, not yet touching, and again notice any change of feeling in your palms. As your hands move closer together, you may begin to feel energy, heat, vibration, or a magnetic pull from your partner's hands. You are experiencing the energy field that surrounds you, the electromagnetic field that is each person's aura. Some people see this field as a color or a light. Others can feel it, even from great distances. Each of you can feel it once you begin to pay attention to it and start developing your sensitivity.

6 Slowly, let your palms meet, feeling the magnetic pull, melding skin on skin, your hands soft and receptive to each other.

7 Hold your contact for several moments. Breathe. Pay attention to your hands and their physical sensations. How does the skin-on-skin contact change the sensation in your hands?

8 After a few breaths, begin to break your contact by moving very slowly apart, as you pass through each other's magnetic field. How far apart can you move and still feel each other?

9 Repeat this exercise two or three times to get the feeling of coming together and departing in this subtle way.

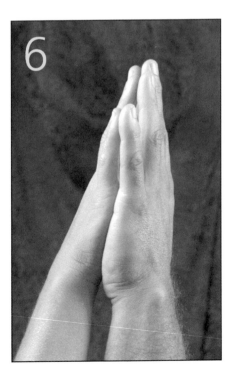

This is an exercise in learning to recognize and respect each other's field and to enter it gently and with awareness. If the giver touches too suddenly without attention, the receiver's body may tighten in protection. The response is automatic and counter to the intention of a massage, which is to relax the body.

scanning your partner's body

This exercise will help develop your awareness and sensitivity as your focus moves from just the hands to the entire body. Often there are visible clues when someone is holding tension in the body. There are also more subtle indications of tension, such as lack of aliveness in the tissue, coolness or heat, color change of the skin, or holding the breath. Sometimes you have an intuitive sense of discomfort or tension in your partner's body. Your touch may be guided there by this sense, and healing can happen through touch that is both loving and sensitive. By practicing this exercise, you can begin to develop this intuitive sense and learn to touch with presence and awareness.

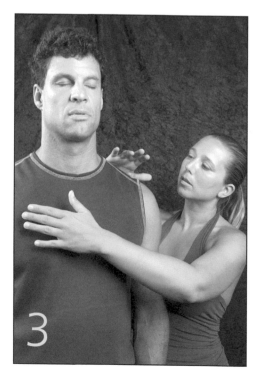

1 Decide who the giver is and who is the receiver, and stand close together but not touching. **Receiver:** close your eyes.

2 Pay attention to your breathing and allow it to be full, without holding your inhalation or exhalation. Breathe all the way down to your belly.

3 **Giver:** Approach your partner and hold one hand several inches from his chest and the other equally close and facing the back. You should be experiencing his energy field in your hands. You can move your hands closer or further away to feel its edges.

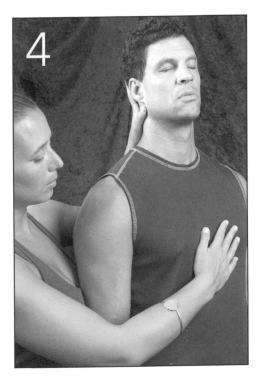

4 After you have made this connection, let your hands pass through this field and slowly touch your partner's back and chest. Let your hands be relaxed, your contact firm and gentle.

5 Hold this connection for several breaths, and as slowly and gracefully as if you were moving through water, let your hands come away from your partner's body.

6 Continue to come in and out of contact in this way all around the body. Observe where you are naturally drawn and let your hands go there. Pay attention to clues. Is your partner holding his breath? Do you notice anything about the color of his skin? Is he obviously holding tension in his muscles, perhaps in the shoulders?

7 Receiver: As your partner comes in and out of contact, bring your awareness to the area being touched and send your breath there. Notice any changes that happen when you do this.

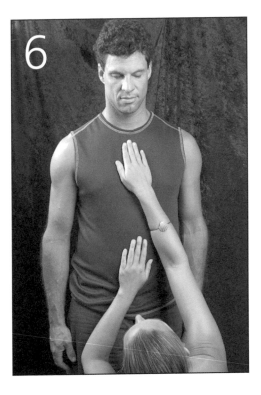

8 **Giver:** After you have scanned and contacted your partner in this way, end by connecting again at the heart, with your hands in front and back of his body, and take a breath together.

9 Break your contact slowly and sensitively.

10 Take your time. The partner who has received the touch will need a few moments to slowly return. **Receiver:** Open your eyes a little at a time. Don't be in a rush to exchange.

11 When you are ready, change places and repeat the exercise.

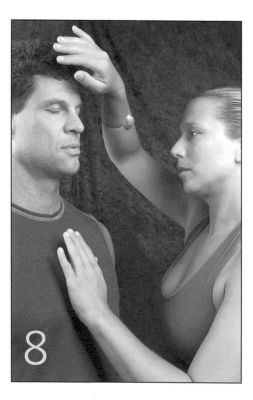

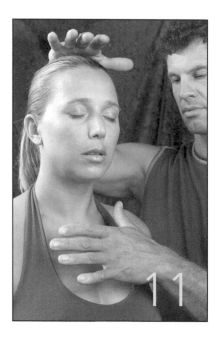

After you both have completed the exercise, spend a few minutes sharing what the experience was like for each of you. You can share what you felt, both in the physical sense and emotionally. Talk about the quality of the touch and ask each other what you liked about being touched in this way. Are there other ways you like to be touched and ways you don't want to be touched?

If your history doesn't include a lot of touch, this exercise may seem strange and unfamiliar, maybe even uncomfortable. I encourage you to stay with it, and enjoy the changes and the healing that can happen through compassionate touch and deep contact.

Listening to Each Other

The gift of being present and listening to each other is one of the joys and benefits of sharing massage. It is not always enough to listen to each other. Your partner wants to know that he has been heard. He needs to feel safe in the knowledge that you will do what he has asked for and not do what makes him uncomfortable. The giver must relinquish any expectations of how the receiver should relax. Rather, meet each other where you are. Agree to be completely honest in your feedback to each other.

This exercise will help you accomplish this communication in the best way.

listening to each other

1 Exchange information about how each of you likes to be touched. Describe the way you like to be touched and the quality of the touch you want to receive. Describe, too, anything you don't particularly like or areas you are not ready to have touched, even by your partner. If either of you has a history of inappropriate

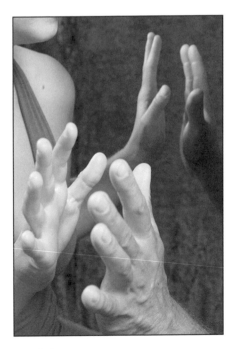

touch, it may take some time to be comfortable with each other in this way. Respect for each other's boundaries will help build a bond of trust between you. Exchange information about where you feel the tension or pain in your body and what kind of touch and pressure you imagine would feel best. Be as specific as you can.

2 Repeat back the information you have heard. That will affirm to your partner that she has been heard. Some of the information you will intuit already from your sense of each other, but you will also need each other's guidance.

It is a good idea to have this conversation before beginning massage, and the communication between you will continue to grow as you connect in this way. It is important as the giver not to let your program or expectation keep you from seeing the receiver's need. Be responsive to your partner's needs and show your love by attending to them. Listening with all your senses is an important skill.

When you are receiving and are communicating feedback to the giver, take care with your language and be positive first. Say "That really feels good," then add what you would like: "and more pressure would feel even better." Be mindful of the words you choose, so as not to hurt each other. Don't make each other wrong; rather, teach each other right!

With the focus on a quiet mind, presence, quality of touch, and thoughtful communication, you are ready to begin the massage.

CHAPTER 2

GIVING & RECEIVING
A MASSAGE

In this chapter, I'll guide you through giving each other a full-body massage. As I suggested earlier, it is a good idea to read the book through once to familiarize yourselves with the concepts and the feeling of the work. After getting a general sense of the massage, try working without the book in front of you. You can always go back and refer to it. Your massage will be more fun for you—and more effective for your partner—if you let yourself feel the work and don't get too caught up in worrying about details. Since there is so much to learn and everyone learns in their own way, find the best way to make this resource work for you so your learning is creative and inspired.

In addition to preparing yourselves as you did in the last chapter, there are a few other things to consider and to communicate about before you begin.

AGREEMENTS

Decide who receives first. Do a complete exchange the first time so you can both have the experience of giving and receiving. At other times, you may want to exchange later.

Decide how much time you want to spend doing the massage. To begin, an hour is good. As your practice develops, your time will naturally expand.

Agree on the music and the lighting.

The receiver makes the decision regarding the drape. The fact that you are a couple doesn't necessarily mean you want to be uncovered during your massage. You can be partially draped, fully draped, or undraped, as long as you're comfortable and warm. A drape can help create a feeling of safety, which is essential to the massage environment.

Decide whether the receiver will start faceup or facedown on the table. Most people like to start facedown, because this position seems less vulnerable and gives you time to get used to being massaged. In addition, the back is where much of the body's tension is held, and thus it is a great place to start.

Agree on how to communicate during the massage. Sound is the perfect way to express your feelings. You can develop a word or hand signal to express your wish for less or more pressure. Always respect the word *stop*.

PREPARATION: GETTING COMFORTABLE

Adjust the height of the massage table before beginning the massage. The best height for the table is at midthigh. The lower the table, the more leverage you have to work with, and the more you must bend your knees and let your thighs support you. A higher table works when you are planning to give a light massage. Try different heights and find what works best for you.

Cover the table with a sheet. Flannel is wonderfully cozy in cold weather, and you can use a heating pad to warm the table first. If you are using the face cradle, cover it with a soft cloth. You can purchase ones made just for this purpose. I suggest you use a bolster or cushion under the receiver's ankles for support. For now, place it on the table with the sheet covering it.

Now invite the receiver to lie facedown on the table. (If your partner prefers to begin faceup, start with the directions for massaging the front of the body.) Cover your partner tenderly with a drape. Adjust the face cradle and bolster to comfortably fit him. Check in with your partner now and make sure he is comfortable. Ask him to make any adjustments he needs to feel comfortable and to feel supported. Both partners take a deep breath.

It is the receiver's responsibility to let your partner know how she is doing, to encourage her, and to direct her to the places that are bothering you the most. It is also good to let her know just how you would like an area worked on. For instance, "Squeeze my shoulder muscles using your fingers and palms," or "Don't put direct pressure there." If it hurts, it is your job to let her know it's too much pressure. There's a good hurt and a bad one. Stay with what feels right to you. Remember, you are the expert on your own body.

Now you are ready to begin the massage. The instructions are for the giver unless otherwise stated.

CORRECT USE OF YOUR BODY

It is essential to learn how to use your body correctly when doing massage. In this way, you don't get tired or sore and don't develop back problems from using your own back incorrectly. There are a few things to remember about good body mechanics.

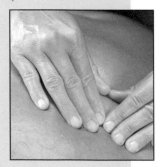

- Stay relaxed and grounded.
- Breathe.
- Drop your center of gravity by bending your knees.
- Use your legs and thighs as your foundation, and always engage them when lifting and moving.
- Keep your back straight as you bend from the waist. Use your legs.
- Relax your shoulders and neck, and straighten your arms for maximum pressure.
- Don't put excessive pressure on your wrists by leaning too heavily on your hands.
- To apply more pressure, use your weight and let the strength come from your legs.
- Don't do anything that will compromise your own physical well-being. By this I mean lifting too much weight or working too hard.
- Remember to dance.

MASSAGING THE BACK OF THE BODY

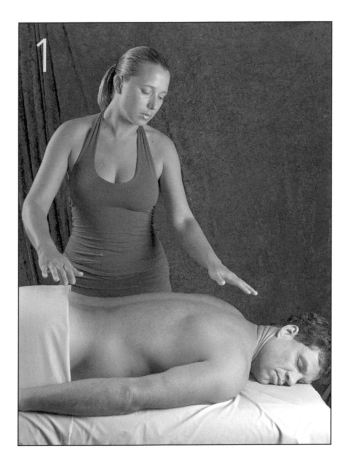

making contact

The initial contact is very important because it sets the tone for the whole massage. When the giver is relaxed and aware, the contact will be sensitive. This will give the receiver the confidence that you are there for him and paying attention to his responses. If you rush in and move quickly, he will naturally tighten up in response. Step back, take a deep breath, and ground yourself. Feel your center. Feel your connection to the earth beneath you. Breathe yourself into the present moment.

1   step next to the table and bring your hands above your partner's body.

2   Let your hands come close to his body, but without touching.

3   As you did in the exercises in chapter 1, feel your partner's energy field. Move around his body, sensing the changes in heat and magnetic attraction as you move from head to toe and back.

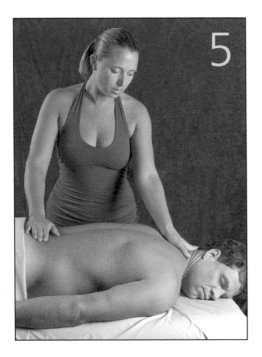

4 Scan the entire field around your partner's body, and then return to the side of the table.

5 Observe your partner's breath. On an inhalation, as your partner's back rises, let your hands gently move through his field and make contact. Let your hands be relaxed and your contact full. Share several moments connected, as you follow the breath, riding its course with your hands resting on your partner's back.

6 Gently break contact, and again move around the table, coming in and out of touch in this way with your partner. Some places will cry out for more pressure, other places for delicate touch. Sense the tissue as you move and apply more or less pressure by leaning your weight onto your hands. Sense beneath the skin and begin to feel muscle, the tendons, the ligaments, the fluids, and finally the bone. Connect with all these levels as you make your way around his body.

7 When you have finished, stand to one side of the table, with one hand on your partner's mid back and one on her lower back, and gently rock your partner on the table. Do this with the same tenderness you would rock a baby. This rhythmic motion is very comforting and settling and will help your partner begin to fall into a deeper state of relaxation. Now you're ready to begin the massage using oil or lotion.

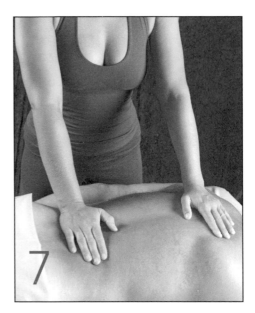

The Back

The back is the place that holds the most tension and does the most work, keeping us erect against the force of gravity. The muscles of the shoulders tighten from any number of causes, from emotional reactions to repetitive motion or patterns of holding tension due to stress. These patterns develop over time and take a long time soften or change. Muscles that are tense can be painful from the contraction itself. Other back problems can arise in the mid back (caused by leaning over) or the lower back (from lifting). Another common trouble spot is between the shoulder blades and the ribs, where those little knotted rhomboid muscles can cause a lot of discomfort. The muscles on either side of the spine get tight and can pull the vertebrae out of alignment. The back needs a lot of care and attention, and it is a great place to start your massage. Your work will move from soft to deep, always returning to soothing strokes that create integration and transition.

Stand at the head of the table, facing your partner. If you're using a drape, fold it down to your partner's hips. Do this with care, since each move you make is part of the massage and sends a message. Every move should be made with the same acute awareness as actual touching.

1 Take a small amount of oil in your palms and rub them together, then bring your hands above your partner's back.

2 Wait as you watch the rise and fall of your partner's breath. On an inhalation, let your hands meet his body. Rest them there, touching, breathing together, connecting in the moment. Don't be in a rush to move into your stroke. Rather, begin to pay attention to what you sense in your hands and in your partner's body.

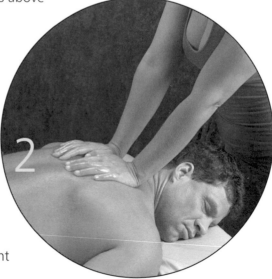

3 Send the message that you are present by being relaxed in stillness together.

4   When you are ready, begin your first massage stroke slowly down your partner's back, one hand on the muscle group on either side of the spine. Begin to lean your weight into your hands as they move down the back, all the way to the *sacrum*, the triangular bone that makes up the base of the spine.

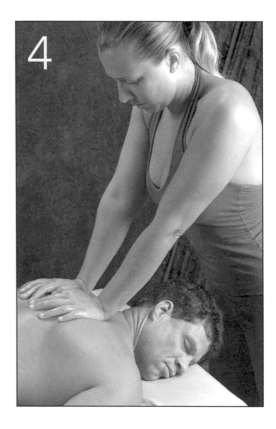

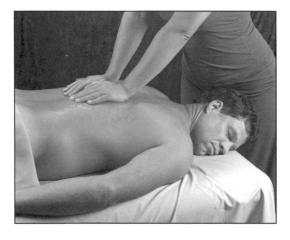

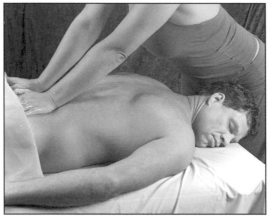

5 Now let your hands continue to the space between the pelvic bone and the hip, making a circle at the hips before bringing your stroke back along the ribs to the shoulders. As you reach the shoulders, cup your hands around the bones, letting your fingers trace the muscles of the shoulders. As you continue, lift the tissue gently, and then follow the curve of the neck to the head.

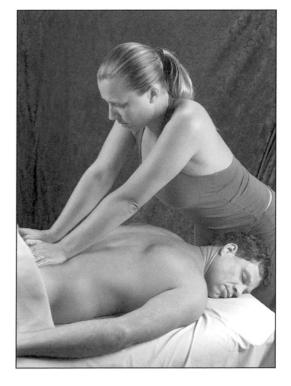

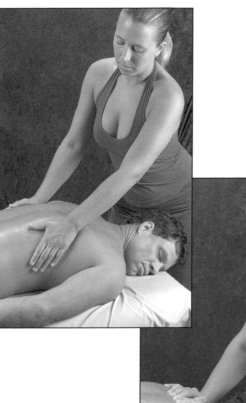

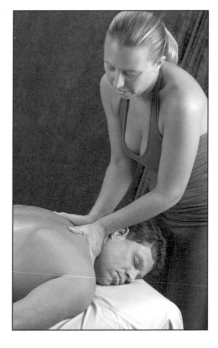

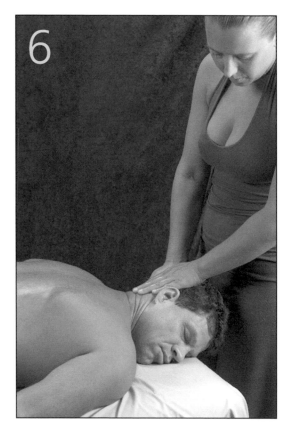

6 Gently complete your stroke at the top of the head by making little circles all over the scalp with your fingertips.

7 Repeat this stroke a few times from the beginning to the end. You will need to add more oil so the back is covered and the skin doesn't pull, but not so much that the skin becomes slippery. Just the right amount will depend on the lubricant and also the skin of both the receiver and the giver.

TRANSITIONS

Transition moves take you from one place on the body to another. They are moves that connect and integrate the work that has gone before and the work that is about to begin. By connecting areas of the body, transitions give the receiver the feeling of wholeness, rather than of lots of little parts. They also help make the giver's journey from one area to the next graceful and flowing, as opposed to choppy and sudden. Transition moves are also used to smooth over areas that have received deep work, such as the shoulders, and prepare the body for where the work is about to begin.

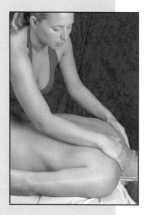

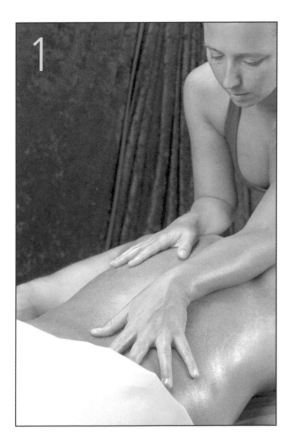

creating variation

1 Alternate your hands moving down the back of your partner's body and shift your weight into one hand, then the other, creating a variation of pressure on the muscles on either side of the spine.

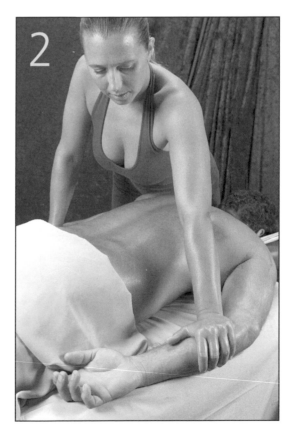

2 Repeat this sequence at least five times to get the feel of the move. Create more variation by changing direction at the shoulder and moving down the arms, gently squeezing the muscles of the arms as you travel to the fingertips. Give the arms a slight pull away from the shoulders as you leave the fingers.

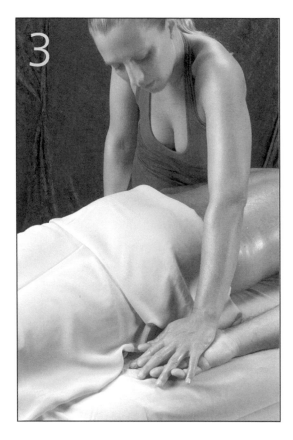

3 Alternate between ending the move at the fingertips and ending at the top of the head. Take your time, and always make sure you complete your move with firm contact; don't drift away at the end of the stroke. If you finish at the head, remember to massage it in a way that is sensual, slow, and loving. By working on the head in this way, you help the receiver to let go of his thoughts and worries and become more settled for his massage. For this reason, some people like to begin the massage by working on the head.

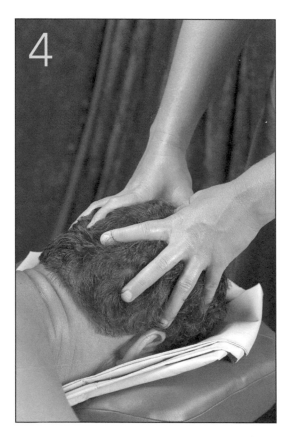

4 Continue to work on the head by making little circles on the scalp, moving it back and forth across the bones of the skull, gently pulling the roots of the hair, combing the hair between your fingers. Let your own body rock gently back and forth as your hands do the work. Stay connected to the rhythmic force that moves you from within. Close your eyes and sense what you are doing. Take your time to complete the head and prepare to transition to the next move.

exploring the bones of the spine

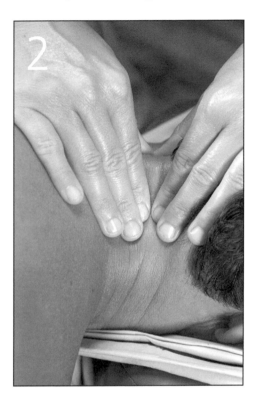

1 Move to the side of the table.

2 Contact the bones of the *cervical spine* (where the neck meets the head) with your fingertips. Gently feel their shape.

3 Being careful not to put direct pressure on the spine, feel the vertebrae of the neck and spine, moving slowly from top to bottom, taking time to explore the shape and movement of the bones.

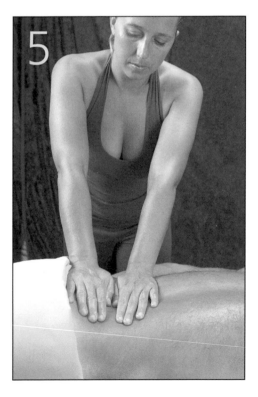

4 With your fingertips, gently move each vertebra from side to side.

5 Continue down the spine to where the spine and ribs attach, and notice the change in the lower back, or *lumbar spine*, where there are no ribs. End at the sacrum. This bone is connected to the other bones that make the pelvic girdle. Rock the sacrum from side to side very gently.

6 Allow one hand to rest on the sacrum. Place the other hand on the mid back, opposite the heart. Let your hands rest there, feeling the rise and fall of the body as the breath moves through. Experience stillness and quiet. Feel your connection to yourself and to your partner.

7 Release your contact and move to the foot of the table, where you will do a long stroke that connects the whole body.

PRESSURE & RHYTHM

Experiment with your pressure by leaning more or less weight into your hands. The strength doesn't come from your hands, but from your body itself. By using your own weight, you create more pressure. Don't be afraid to lean your weight onto your hands if your partner asks for more pressure. Add pressure gradually, never suddenly. Always release pressure on the receiver's inhalation and apply pressure on an exhalation. That way you are working together, rather than in opposition to each other. As you increase your pressure and go deeper, go a little slower. The receiver's body opens gradually and responds to a gentle invitation to expand and find balance.

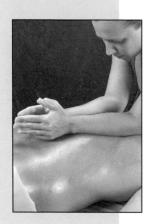

When you repeat this opening stroke, which becomes long and graceful with practice, a rhythm or pattern of movement begins to emerge from a feeling inside. As you find your groove, drawing on your own sense of timing and movement, you can expect to move into an altered state where your mind is at ease and you feel at home in your own body. Repetition of the opening stroke also helps the receiver sink more readily into a relaxed state. The rhythm of your heartbeat, the rhythm of your own breath, the rhythm of your movement, of music or external sounds like the ocean, all help to relax the body/mind. For the giver, this rhythm frames the work. Once you have connected to your partner and to this rhythm, the connection remains, even though you take your hands off the receiver's body from time to time.

the long stroke

The long stroke connects the body from the tips of the toes to the tips of the fingers. It integrates the work, giving the receiver the feeling of wholeness and of all his parts being connected and elongated. It is used to travel from one area of the body to another, and if done well, it is a wonderfully delicious stroke to receive. It takes some practice to get it smooth and flowing. The key is learning to move with your stroke, to keep up with your hands so there is no starting or stopping. Rather, it is one long, continuous, flowing stroke that feels like the motion of a rolling wave or a long, slow, deep breath.

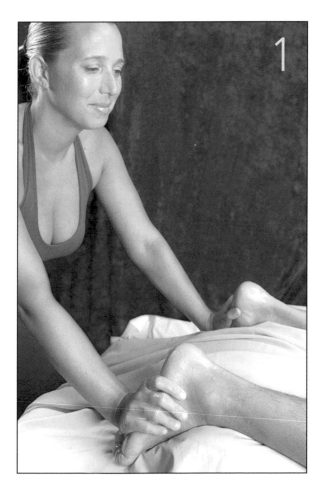

1 Apply oil to your palms. Approach the feet with the same loving care you did the back. Let your hands rest on your partner's feet, holding them gently. Feel your own feet connected to the ground beneath you.

2 Take some more oil in your hands, move to the side of the table, and begin a long stroke up the back of both legs, one hand on each leg. Go all the way to the top of the leg, circle the buttocks and hips, and bring your stroke back down the legs, again creating a circular path of motion.

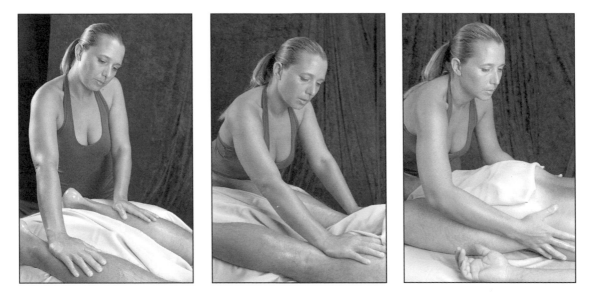

3 After two or three repetitions, you can continue the long stroke all the way up the back, around the shoulders, and down the arms, hands, and fingertips. As you come down the arms, gently squeeze the muscles of the arms and give the wrists a gentle pull to encourage the shoulders to release before letting go at the fingertips.

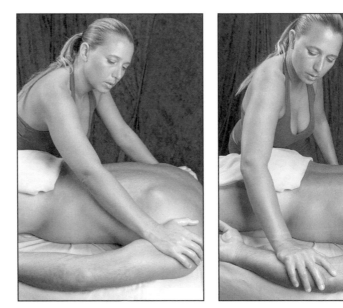

4 When you reach the fingertips, come back to the foot of the table, apply more oil as needed, and repeat this move several times, spreading the oil evenly over the tops and sides of the legs. Move slowly along the side of the table to keep up with your hands.

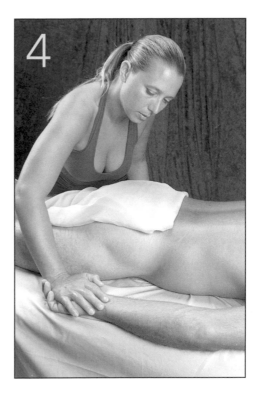

5 Repeat this long connecting stroke two or three times to develop a feel for the move. You'll find you will enjoy your own movement as you travel your partner's body. Feel pleasure in the dance of your fingers as they stroke your partner's skin, offering support, love, and healing intention. This nurturing and healing flows from your heart right through to your hands to your loved one's body.

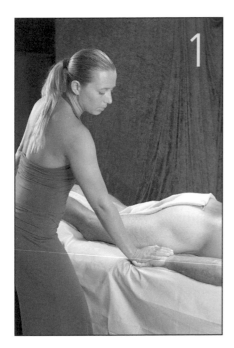

A variation of the long stroke that also connects the upper and lower body can be done by moving to the side of the table and facing your partner's body. This is an integrating move, fun both to do and to receive.

1 Place both hands together at the hip. Bend your knees, dropping your center of gravity.

2 Now move your hands in opposite directions, one hand along the rib cage to the arm and hand, the other down the thigh to rest on the foot. If you can't reach, you can begin the same way and choose to either move up the body toward the head or move down the leg to the foot.

3 Repeat on the other side.

These long strokes are the skeleton of the massage, and details are filled in around these repeated moves. With practice, these strokes will become smooth, and you will begin to add detail that will come to you intuitively when you begin to trust yourself in this practice. Before continuing on, check in with your partner to see how he is doing. Keep the conversation to a minimum so as not to break the sweetness of the mood you have created.

THE IMPORTANCE OF FEEDBACK

Ask for specific feedback about pressure, about the way you're using your palms or fingers, and about the pace of your work. There are obvious clues in the body to look for that indicate discomfort. These are holding the breath, clenching the jaw, sudden movement, or tightening the muscles in response to touch. If you see any of these, it is important to stop and ask for feedback. Something may have been triggered that has nothing to do with the moment or with you. It is possible that an old memory or a fear has intruded and caused your partner to tense up in response. Feedback is essential here, so there is no misunderstanding as to what is going on. If a difficult moment arises for the receiver, the 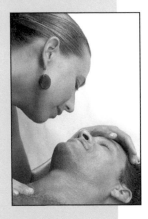 giver can be supportive by being there in a loving way, without judgment. Remember too that feedback is not meant to be critical but helpful. The receiver can help by being positive and specific: "I liked the long strokes on my arms, but the deep pressure on my shoulder is a little uncomfortable. With less pressure, it would feel better."

The Shoulders

For many of us, our shoulders carry the weight of the world. We tend to raise them up toward our ears for protection; to round them, closing off the possibility of full breath; and to hold them immobile, eventually causing great discomfort. The shoulder or *trapezius* muscles need to be coaxed back to their natural relaxed state, where they more effectively support you and help you move. After years of holding tension, the muscles become rigid and sometimes are very sensitive to the touch. For this reason, it is very important to check in often with your partner when working here.

1 Go to the side of the table and face your partner's head. Gently lift his arm and place it on your thigh, as you sit on the corner of the table. You are now in a comfortable position to address the shoulders and at the same time give your legs a rest by sitting for a few minutes. Put some oil on your hands if you need the lubrication, but don't make the shoulders too slippery.

2 Notice if there is any tension in your partner's shoulders. Do they feel hard or tight to the touch? Did your partner give you any information about his shoulders? Approach them softly and increase your pressure as needed. Begin to knead the muscles of the shoulders using your palms and your fingers. Gently work the muscles from front to back and lightly squeeze them to increase the circulation there. Fresh blood brings needed oxygen to muscles, and this in turn helps them relax.

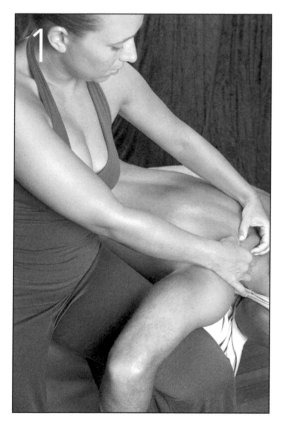

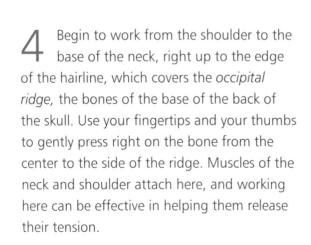

3 Experiment with using different parts of your hands to massage the muscles. The palms are good for broader work, whereas the fingertips are best for small areas and refined work.

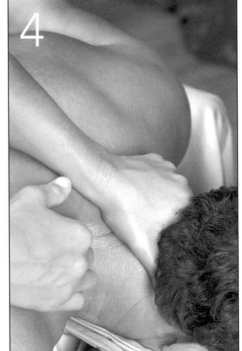

4 Begin to work from the shoulder to the base of the neck, right up to the edge of the hairline, which covers the *occipital ridge,* the bones of the base of the back of the skull. Use your fingertips and your thumbs to gently press right on the bone from the center to the side of the ridge. Muscles of the neck and shoulder attach here, and working here can be effective in helping them release their tension.

5 Work your way up onto your partner's scalp, lovingly massaging his
head. Move the scalp back and forth across
the bones. Comb your partner's hair with
your fingers. Take your time here and make
your work sensuous and slow.

6 Before completing the work on the
shoulder, reach one hand across to
the other shoulder and knead them both
together. Notice the difference in the way
the muscles feel on each side. Most people
favor one side or hold more tension on one
side than the other, and that side often ap-
preciates deeper work in order to release.

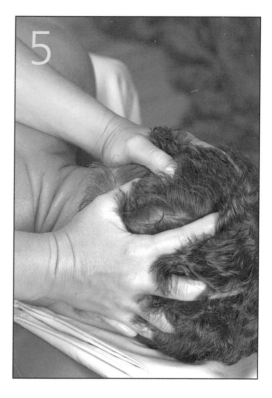

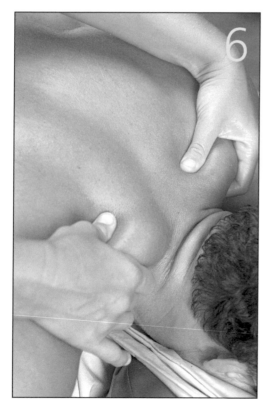

7 After you have spent a few minutes
massaging the shoulders and neck,
you can make a smooth transition back to
standing by lifting the shoulder as you get
up from the table and then, supporting the
elbow and shoulder, return the arm to its
resting place on the table. Prepare for the
next move, the shoulder blades.

The Shoulder Blades

The shoulder blades are another place we hold tension. This is experienced by the receiver as if there are little knots in the tissue, and the shoulders may be stiff and tight and not able to complete their full range of motion. How deep you work on the muscles around the shoulder blades will depend on the receiver's request. The deeper into the tissue you go, the slower you must go, always working with your partner's breath. If he needs more pressure in a specific spot, ask him to take a deep breath, and as he exhales, add more pressure to your move. As he inhales again, lighten your pressure. Move in and out of depth with the breath. Never work against the breath. This is one of the few rules in this practice, and working on the shoulder blades will be easier if you follow this guideline.

1 Come to the side of the table and face your partner's head.

2 Gently cup the shoulder in your outside hand, lean forward, and rest your elbow and forearm on the table.

3 Take a wide-leg stance, or lunge position, so you have a broad base of support.

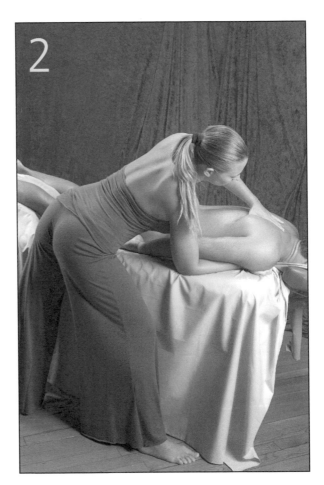

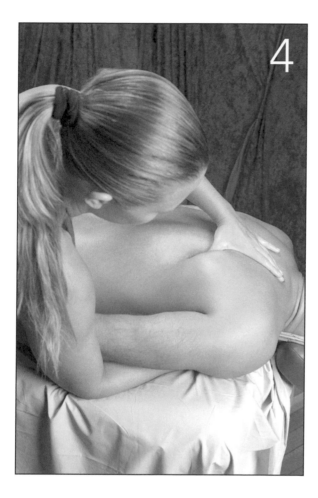

4 With your other hand, trace the *scapula*, or wing bone, starting at the bottom and working your way up to the top of the bone. Gently rub the knots against the rib bones, and be sure to check with your partner to see how he feels. An open scapula will allow your fingers to slip between the ribs and scapula, where you can access deeper layers of muscle. Work up and down the area, using your fingertips to explore the tissue there.

5 Examine the movement of the shoulder by supporting the shoulder in your hands and moving it in small rotations, both forward and back.

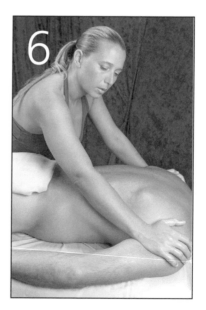

6 Transition from the shoulder blade with some softer strokes connecting the entire back. Move down to the hips and lower back.

The Low Back

Tension and compression often settle in the lower back, around the lumbar region, where the spine is without the support of the ribs, and the *sacral region,* the bottom of the spine. There are many reasons for this, the obvious one being that we are erect creatures in a gravity field that is constantly pulling on us. If we stand all day, after eight hours there is bound to be some compression in the spine. Stretching, movement, and elongation can relieve this, but for many people, lack of movement compounds the compression. Lifting and carrying can also contribute to pain in this area.

If the pain is severe, it will often respond to cold and heat, applied alternately. Stretching and elongating the spine, as well as massaging around the sacrum and the *sacroiliac joints* (the union of the *ileum,* or hip bone, and the sacrum) and the hips, can help relieve discomfort in the lower back. If compression is severe and lying facedown on the table is a problem, try using a pillow under the hips to elevate them; that takes some pressure off of the spine.

Another possible cause of discomfort in the sacral region is the release of hormones in premenstrual women. Many women suffer from this, and while stretching helps, they will often request counterpressure against the bones.

PREMENSTRUAL DISCOMFORT

Some women suffer from hormonal changes that create discomfort in the sacral region of the lower back. I was one of those women. Each month, I would get sore in that area, and no amount of stretching or soaking in warm water relieved the pressure. The only thing that felt good to me was *counterpressure,* pressure directly on the sacrum and downward toward the legs.

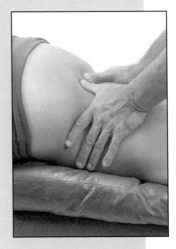

Women are often bloated and uncomfortable during their premenstrual days and can be crabby without much provocation. A sweet massage could help relieve some of the anxiety that can go with that. Go gently on the belly, and remember the breasts may be tender as well.

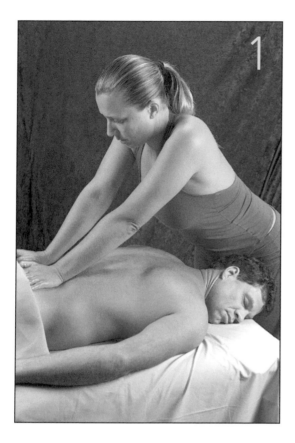

1 Begin a long stroke down the back, and when you reach the sacrum, lean your weight into your hands and give a gentle thrust toward the feet to elongate the spine. Imagine your moves opening the area, bringing more breath and movement to the lower back, extending the spine, and opening the hips.

2 With your palms, rock the sacrum gently from side to side to explore its movement.

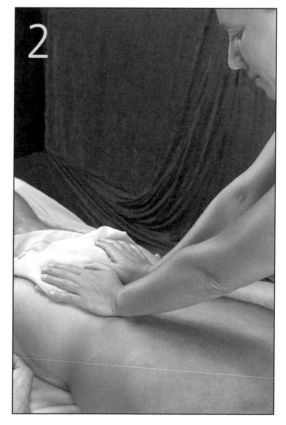

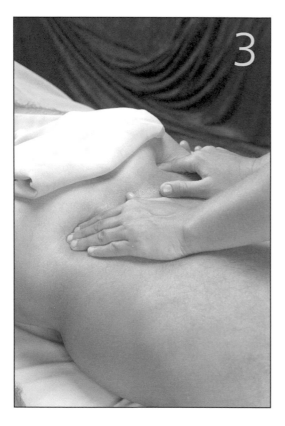

3 Use your fingertips to work right on the top of the sacrum itself, making little circles and moving out toward the sacroiliac joint.

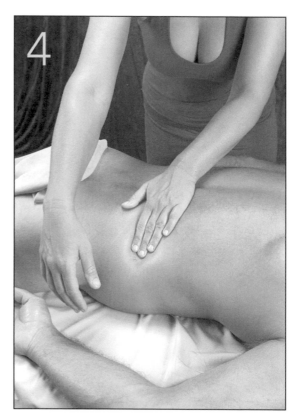

4 Include the hip muscles by working your fingers into the soft tissue between the hip bone and the head of the thigh bone. Tight muscles in this area can contribute to tension in the lower back.

Between these focused areas of work, always return to your long strokes to connect the areas of attention and bring a sense of wholeness to the body. These are the moves that feel so nurturing and give your partner the feeling of being cherished and held by you. Remember the dance. Remember to relax and enjoy the gift of giving. Never hesitate to stop and be still, to hold a hand or a foot or let your hands rest gently on the head, allowing the silence to speak.

The Ribs

Working on the ribs is beneficial for the receiver in that it encourages the breath. Many people don't breathe fully, and this work can help invite deeper breathing, which is so central to the way of massage. Even the sound of the giver's breath encourages the breath and relaxation of the receiver.

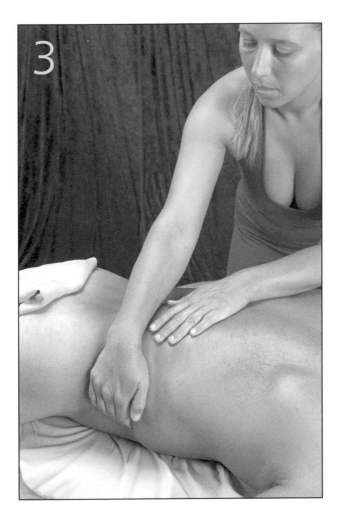

1 Go to one side of the table and oil your hands.

2 Bend your knees and bring your hands slowly into contact with your partner's ribs on the opposite side of the body from where you're standing.

3 Alternately and rhythmically move your hands across his ribs, gently pulling toward you.

4 Let your fingers explore the spaces between the ribs as well as the rib cage, and lightly massage the muscles there.

5 Go to the opposite side and repeat this, moving up and down the rib cage.

6 Notice any changes that have happened. Perhaps there was a spontaneous breath or a deep sigh. Complete with a long transition stroke that covers the whole back and ends at the feet. This is where you'll work next.

connecting the upper & lower body

The way to connect the upper body with the lower body is to use the long stroke that begins at the feet and ends at the fingertips or top of the head. You can do this as you begin and end the work on the feet and legs. You can add it anywhere in between and repeat it as many times as you want. A few repetitions of most moves are better than just one or two. The body needs time to transition and integrate, and it responds well to moves that are repeated.

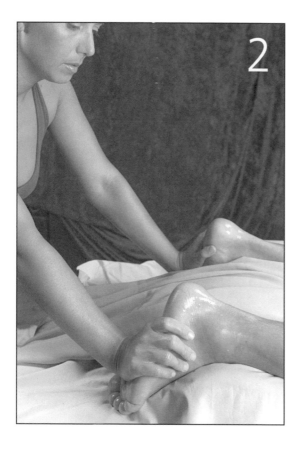

1 Move to the foot of the table. Put some oil in your palms.

2 Rest your palms on your partner's soles. Take a moment to reconnect to your own breath and to that of your partner.

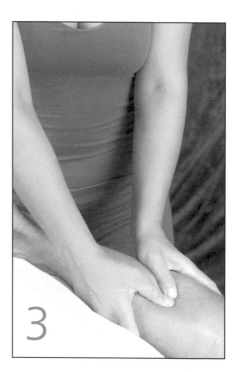

3 With both hands on one leg, beginning at the foot, start a long stroke up the back of the leg.

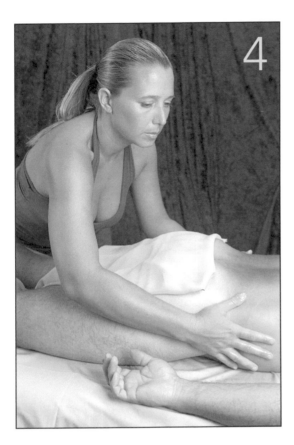

4 When you reach the hip, spread your hands and begin your return down the sides and back of the leg. You may need to apply more oil as you move up the leg.

5 Repeat this several times. Lean your body weight easily into your hands so as to apply more pressure to the thighs. There is greater muscle mass here, and additional pressure is needed to work this area effectively. If the stretch is too long to reach the hip, move to the side of the table so you can reach all the way as you move up the leg and back. Attempt to keep your movement smooth and even. This takes some practice, so give yourself time to get comfortable with the moves.

6 Imagine moving with the grace of a dancer and the groundedness of a martial artist. You will enjoy the practice more if you fully engage yourself.

7 Now begin at the feet and take your stroke all the way up the body and down the arms, saying goodbye at the fingertips.

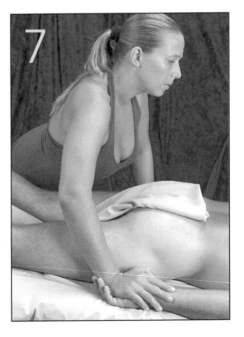

As you struggle with trying to remember the moves, be kind to yourself. It takes time and practice to learn each technique. Remember that this work is as natural to you as is the need to touch and be touched. When love is expressed through your touch, it gives your technique both meaning and depth. Technique alone is empty. Try not to get stuck there. Give your brain a rest by closing your eyes and just feeling the work.

The Feet

Now that you have connected the body from toes to fingers, you are ready to work on the feet. For people who spend their days standing a lot, you can bet there will be some tired and grateful feet to rub. We will include the feet in the full-body massage. Chapter 3 will examine foot massage further, as a form in itself.

REFLEXOLOGY

There is a school of massage called *reflexology* where the entire treatment focuses on the feet. Reflexologists believe that the soles of the feet contain specific pressure points that correspond to organs, muscles, and nerves of the entire body. Calcium deposits can form as little crystals at these points. By working the crystals loose for the body to reabsorb, you are directly affecting other places in the body. Reflexology is also used to diagnose illness, by indicating where trouble may be on the inside as it corresponds to the reflex point on the foot. The foot is read as if a map of the body were superimposed over it. The arch of the foot corresponds to the spine, the upper and lower body are divided by the center of the foot, and so on. If you are interested in studying reflexology further, I recommend Deborah Ardell Hill's book, *Spiritual Reflexology: Spiritual Gifts of the Body* (1999, DAH Enterprises).

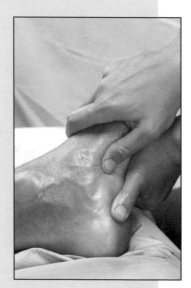

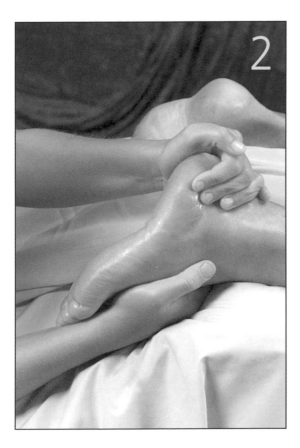

1 Go to the foot of the table.

2 Gently lift and stretch the foot while you sit on the end of the table or on a stool at the foot of the table. Cradle your partner's foot on your lap.

3 Apply oil to your hands and spread it evenly over the sole of the foot.

4 Using your palms and your thumbs, rub the foot firmly, squeezing and gently stretching the foot away from the body. Make sure your touch is firm so as to avoid any ticklishness. Remember, we walk on these feet all day, and they can take a lot of pressure.

5 Trace the valleys between the bones and tendons on the feet with your fingertips.

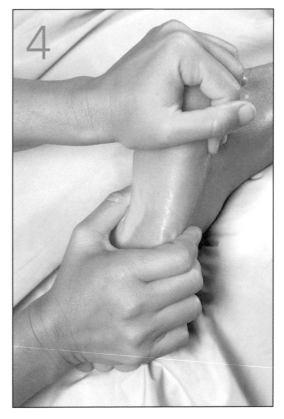

6 Spread the pad, or ball, of the foot by leaning into it and pressing and opening the spaces between the bones.

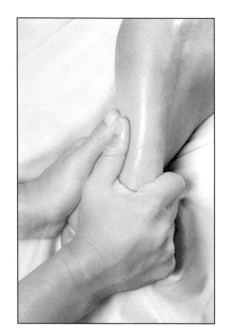
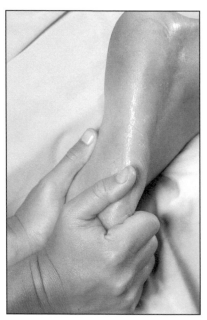

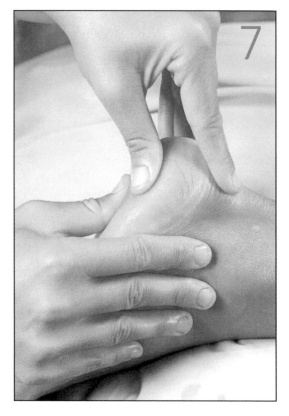

7 Cradle the heel and work the instep from the heel to the ball of the foot.

8 Use your fingers to make little circles along the sole of the foot while pressing into the ball of the foot.

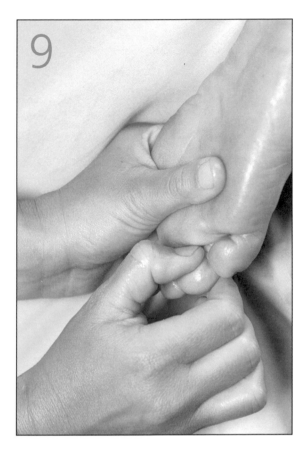

9 Massage each toe, pulling gently to create space between the joints. Rotate each toe lovingly, and gently squeeze the nail as you come off the tip of the toe.

10 Rotate the ankle and massage the Achilles tendon, which connects the muscles of the back of the leg to the heel of the foot.

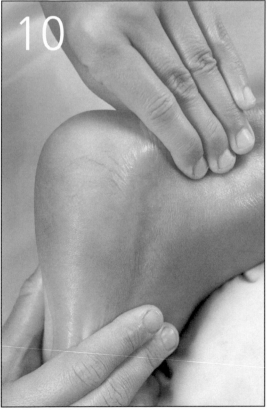

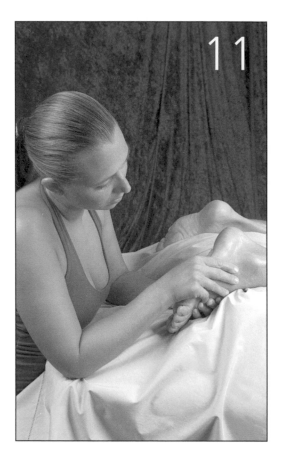

11 Rub the entire foot, leaning into your moves for additional pressure as needed.

12 Close your eyes and let yourself just feel it from within and get lost in the work you're doing. Take your time and explore the feet as if you are discovering their magic for the first time. Find ways to open the foot by moving the bones around as you explore all its possible movements. Glide your fingers between the toes and before leaving, make sure you don't leave one lonely part of the foot untouched.

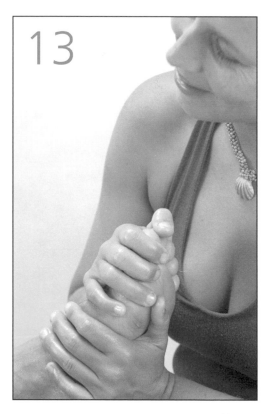

13 Complete the work by cradling the foot between your hands and just holding it for a moment or two. Return the foot to the table. After working on the other foot, prepare to stand to massage the legs.

The Lower Leg

To massage the legs, you will need to stand balanced at the end of the table. The lower leg can best be worked on with fingers or palms. Before working on the lower leg, do one long stroke to connect the work you completed on the foot to the work you're about to do on the legs.

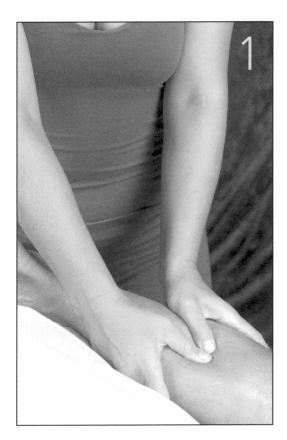

1 The calves have a two-headed muscle that has a clear split in the center. Define each head of it with your fingers, pressing lightly in the center where the two meet.

2 Work along the grain of the muscle with your fingertips and then your palms.

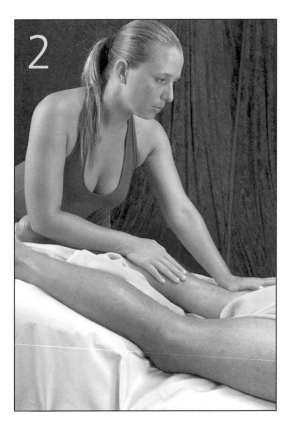

3 Work across the grain of the muscles, kneading it as you move from the ankle to the knee.

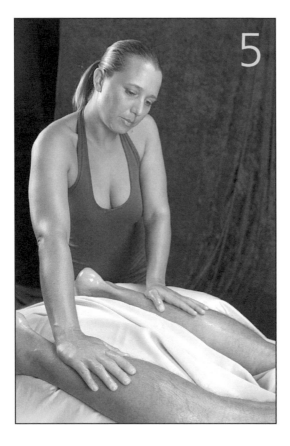

4 Check with your partner regarding pressure. Some people are very sensitive in the area of the calf, so it is best to work lightly at first to see what pressure he prefers.

5 If the receiver is a runner with highly developed calf muscles, he may respond to broader and deeper pressure.

CREATING THE SENSE OF A THREE-DIMENSIONAL BODY

When you're working on the legs (or the arms, for that matter), you want to give your partner the sense of a three-dimensional leg, rather than a top and bottom leg. To accomplish this, on the return from the long stroke, let your hands move along the sides of the thighs and under the knees and along the front of the leg on the way to the foot.

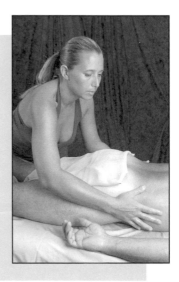

The Thighs

When working on the thighs, you can apply more pressure by using your palms or even your forearms. The muscles of the thighs are broad and respond to a wide, firm pressure. You can work either with the grain of the muscle or across it. It's often effective to do both.

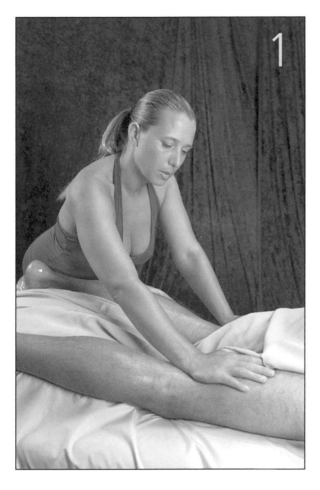

1   Lean into your hands as you apply more oil to the thigh.

2   The hamstrings are a strong muscle group, and some people will need more pressure than you can get in your hands. In that case, use your forearms and apply more weight to them. Alternate stroking from one arm to the other. Be sure to bend your knees and drop your center of gravity so as not to strain your back.

3   Working lightly at the knee, move up the leg by kneading the muscles from side to side with your fingers and more deeply with your palms.

4   Trace the hamstrings to their attachment at the sit bone, which can be found in the center of the top of the thigh.

5   Now, with an open palm, work up the entire leg to the hip. When you reach the hip, slide one hand to the front of the leg so the leg is supported front and back. Now, lean back and come down the leg with opposing hands, giving a light tug on the leg to elongate and open the joint of the hip. This three-dimensional move feels whole and supportive. You add the traction by simply leaning back

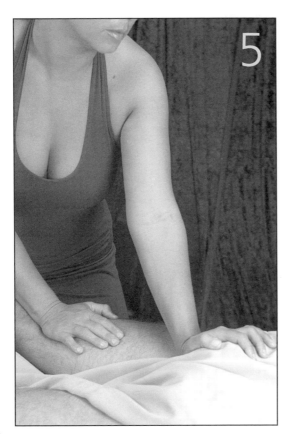

5

as you move. Do these moves only if it doesn't strain your back. If your partner's leg is very heavy, do a variation of the move without lifting the leg.

6 Repeat your long strokes, first on the leg only, then taking it all the way up the back and down the arm to the hand. Hold the hand in yours for a moment before gently releasing your partner.

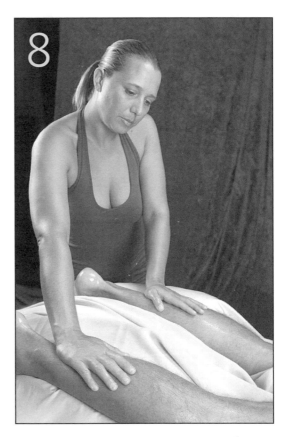

8

7 Before moving to the other leg, quietly check in with your partner for feedback regarding pressure on the leg. This feedback must be continual throughout the massage, if not in words, then in sounds or expressions.

8 Now move to the other foot and repeat the work you did on the first foot and leg. Take your time and match your moves, so both legs and feet feel evenly attended to.

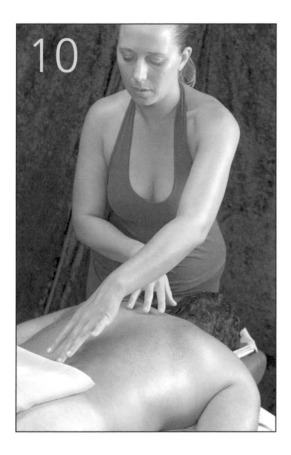

9 Integrate the work on both legs by starting with a hand holding each foot. After a breath or more, do a finishing long stroke including the legs and back, around the shoulders, and down the arms to the hands, where your palms rest together in a moment of appreciation for each other.

10 Do a series of feather-light strokes up the spine before coming away slowly and returning to the side of the table to close.

finishing the back of the body

It's important to bring closure to your massage so your partner is not left wondering what's next or where you have gone. Part of this ending is the long connecting strokes over the whole body, done in a slow and sensuous way. It is best to end in stillness, allowing time for integration. You can follow the instructions below or come up with you own way of ending. Just make sure it is clear.

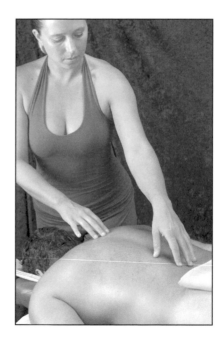

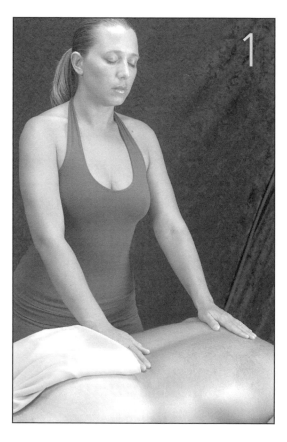

1 Follow your partner's breath and as his body rises to meet you, quietly place your palms on his back, one hand in the mid back opposite the heart, the other on the sacrum.

2 Rest there. Take your time. Let your breathing fall together as you connect on this primal level. You both may feel bathed in calm and feel that your heart is open. Knowing your partner's vulnerabilities and pain helps you feel more compassion for each other. Feeling this compassion helps each other heal.

3 Cover your partner with a drape to keep him warm as you slowly step away.

4 Take some deep breaths and stretch yourself, allowing your body to expand and open. Reconnect with yourself. Notice any subtle shifts or changes in your own energy.

5 Drink some water and bring some to your partner. Keep your voices low so as not to break the peaceful feeling. Ask your partner to turn over.

6 Remove the pillow from under the ankles. Assist your partner in turning over and cover him as desired. Ask him if he needs anything before you begin the front side of the body. Make your transition nice and slow.

MASSAGING THE FRONT OF THE BODY

The receiver is now lying on the table faceup. The giver can remove the bolster and face cradle from its holder. Place the bolster under the knees by lifting and supporting the legs while you slide the cushion under the sheet. Make sure your partner is comfortable and warm, and offer an eye pillow. Sometimes people feel cool when they first turn over, so have a warm cover nearby.

VULNERABILITY & TRUST

Lying faceup on the table is a vulnerable position. Even if modesty is not usually an issue, a drape may help the receiver feel comfortable and address

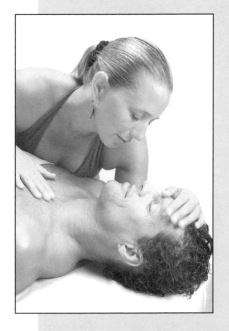

the psychological need to feel a bit protected in this supine position. There are also issues of trust that come up for people on the table faceup. If there is a history of abuse, it may be difficult to trust even your spouse. Memories may be stirred by the situation. Sometimes people will involuntarily relive bad memories, and fear will start to build. If this is the case for your partner, your loving presence and the reminder that you are there together and it's safe in the present moment will often help to bring him back. Encourage your partner to breathe and to maintain eye contact with you. Be there for him in the most loving way you can, and keep encouraging him to return to the present and not let his mind return to traumatic times. Take all the time needed to make sure he is comfortable and ready before you begin.

making contact on the front side of the body

As the giver, prepare yourself by taking a moment to breathe fully and bring your attention back to your center. Ground yourself by connecting to the earth that supports you, while receiving energy from deep in its core. Let that energy rise up through your body and into your hands through the conscious use of your breath. As this energy begins to fill you, step closer to the side of the table and watch your partner's breathing. His stomach should be soft on an inhalation, and you will see it rise and expand. Deep breathing is done with the belly expanding as you take a deep breath. Exhalation can be long and slow, matching the inhalation as the lungs contract and all the air is forced out. When you breathe deeply, you are closer to your feelings; the breath takes you to your core. Deep breathing is the most integral part of the process of relaxing. Letting go is done through breath, and the bodymind follows.

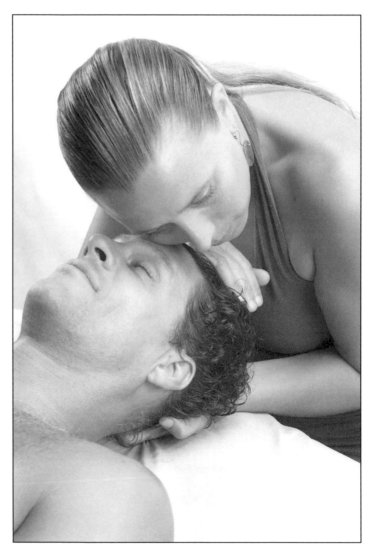

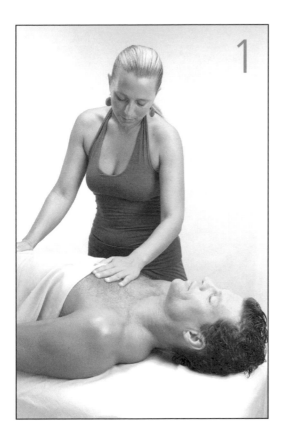

1 Observe your partner's breath and let your hands begin to pass through his energy field, connecting to his body on an inhalation. Let his body and your hands almost breathe together as they connect. Let one hand rest on your partner's upper chest and the other on his belly, just below the navel. Let your hands be soft and your contact full, and take some time to breathe together, feeling the energy flow between you.

2 Breathe your love into your partner's body. Receive his through his breath.

3 After a few moments of connecting, come away as gently as you entered and return to the head of the massage table.

the long stroke on the front of the body

This circular stroke is similar to the one done on the back of the body. It is used in both the beginning and the end of the massage. This stroke integrates the front of the upper body and addresses the spine by gently elongating it. It also encourages breath by engaging the belly and ribs.

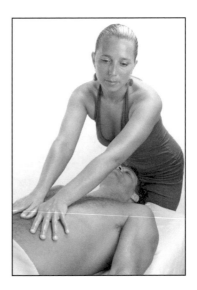

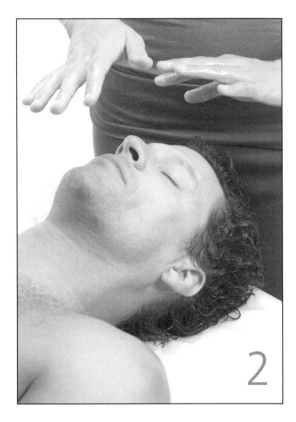

1 Go to the head of the table.

2 In preparation for your first long stroke on the front of the body, fold the drape down to your partner's hips. Then apply some oil to your hands. If you are using aromatherapy or scented oils, circle the scent a few inches above his nose so he can enjoy the fragrance as he inhales deeply.

3 Take a moment to center yourself again before making your first contact on the chest. Come through your partner's energy field and softly rest your hands on his chest. Take a moment to connect here before beginning your first long stroke down the front of the body.

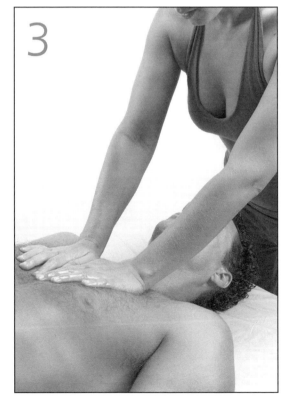

4 Lean softly into your hands as you move down the chest and belly to the hips. Less pressure is needed on the front of the body, so be mindful of not using too much weight or compressing the chest.

5 Circle the hips, come back up the side of the body, and lift the ribs slightly to encourage breath, as you shift your weight and lean back a little.

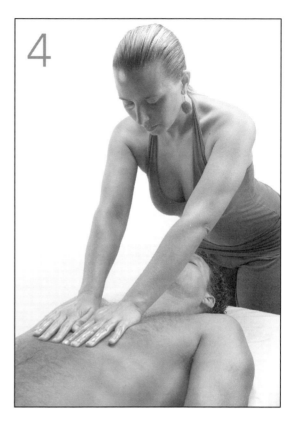

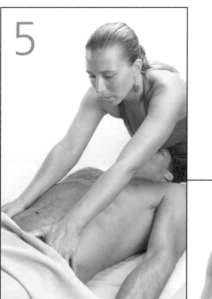

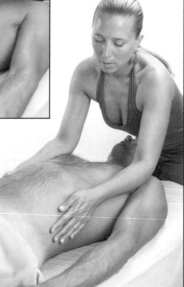

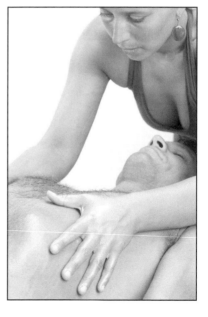

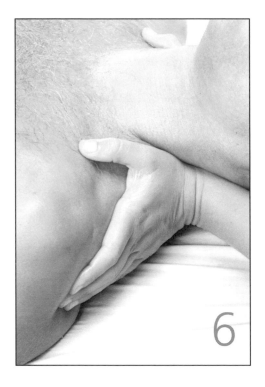

6 Continue your stroke around the shoulder and up the back of the neck, ending with a gentle lift of the head. Bring your hands gracefully away from the crown of the head.

Practice this stroke by repeating it several times, allowing yourself to fall into your rhythm, shifting your body weight and leaning in and out of your stroke. Notice any changes in breath. Your breath will be faster than your partner's because you're moving and he is still. You can stop at any time, anywhere, and reconnect to each other's breath, pausing for integration while your hands rest silently on the body. Work slowly and be patient with yourself as you practice this move. It takes time to feel comfortable with it, and each time you do it will be a bit smoother and easier.

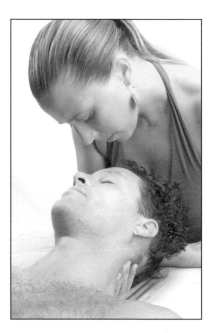

The Neck

The transition from the long stroke to the neck is easy and natural. As you come off the top of the head, take a few moments to massage the scalp. Comb your fingers through your partner's hair and gently pull it at the roots. Now you're ready to work on the neck.

If you have a stool, you can sit at the head of the table rather than stand. Another way to work on your partner's neck and head is to have him slide down the table toward his feet, giving enough room at the head of the table for you to sit. Your partner's head can rest between your legs. This position brings more intimacy to the moment and is comfortable for the giver.

1 When you are comfortably seated, connect with your partner's head in the same soft way you have before. Let you hands rest a moment before making any move at all.

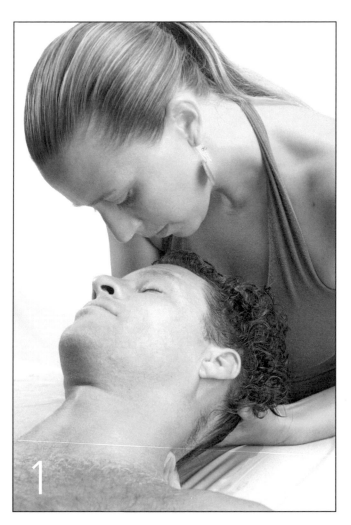

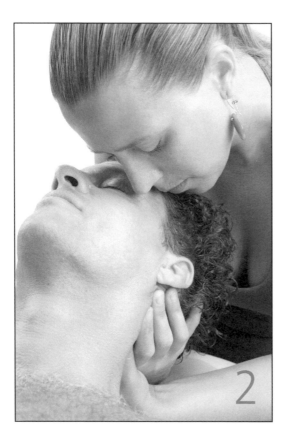

2 Wrap your hands around his head in a way that fully supports it and slowly begin to lift it an inch or two off the table.

3 Fully support the head. If your partner is not holding up his own head, the weight of the head should feel quite heavy in your hands. If he is holding, encourage him to let go by giving you the weight of his head.

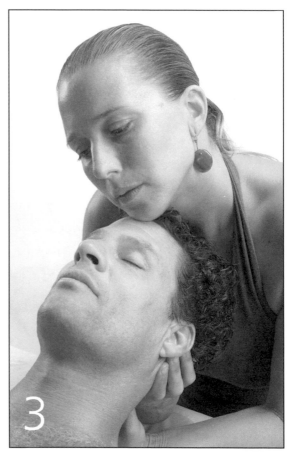

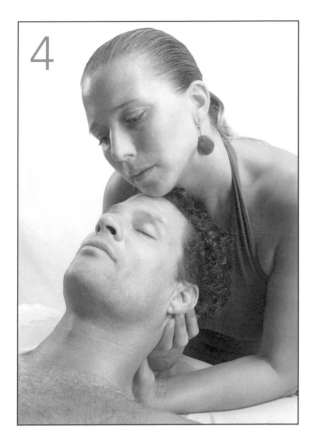

4 Little by little, explore the range of motion in the neck by bringing his chin closer to his chest as you gently lift the head.

5 Lift until you feel some resistance, and then slowly bring the head back to rest on the table.

6 With both hands supporting the head, turn it slowly to the left and to the right. Working slowly gives your partner the time to adjust and make the internal changes necessary to let go. It also helps him become aware of where he is holding tension. Begin to work toward his full range of motion.

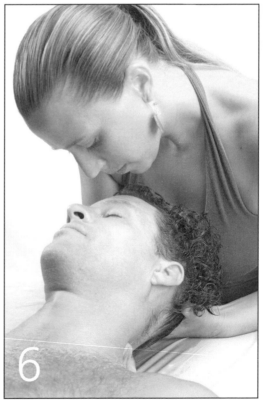

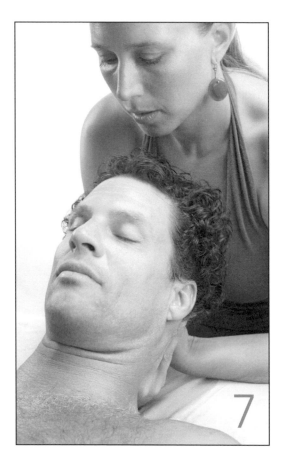

7 Lift the head once more so that there is enough room for your hand to fit under it to massage the muscles of the neck. With one hand supporting the neck, the other hand is free to massage the small muscles on either side of the cervical spine.

8 Gently squeeze the muscles with your fingertips and make little circles as you go from the base of the neck to the head and back again. If he is holding, encourage him to let go by giving you the weight of his head.

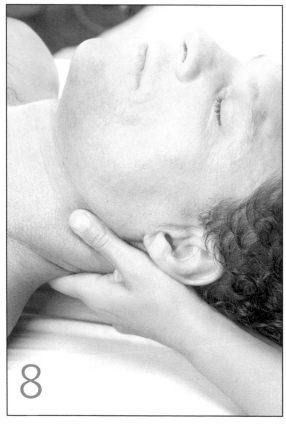

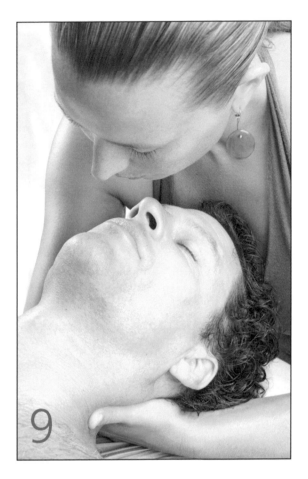

9 Use your palms to caress your partner's neck, elongating it and inviting the muscles to let go.

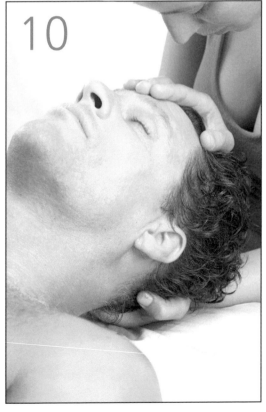

10 Complete your work here by bringing the head down gently to the table. Continue to cradle your partner's head in your palms with as much tenderness as you would a baby or child.

11 After several breaths, slide your hand out from under the head and let your upper hand lift up from the forehead.

The Head
You can remain seated to work on the head. This is a good time to close your eyes and let yourself go with the feeling of what you're doing, rather than depending on visual information. Since you don't have to move, it is a safe time for this type of exploration. Some people prefer to not have too much oil in their hair, and since the face has its own oil, you need just a little when working there. The *oohs* and *ahhs* will let you know just how much they appreciate the work on the head.

1   Begin by massaging the scalp. Circular moves with your fingertips all over the scalp can create a hypnotic trance for your loved one.

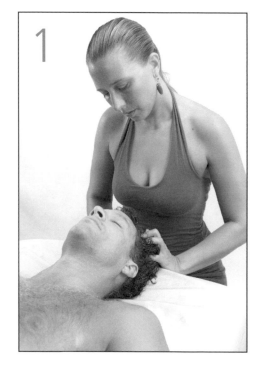

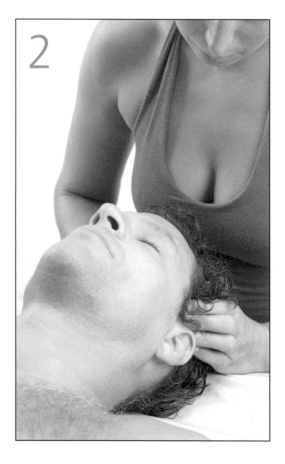

2   Explore the bones of the head, noticing their shape and their valleys and protrusions. Continue to use your fingertips. Let your whole body rock slightly back and forth as you work. This barely detectable motion gives depth, dimension, and rhythm to your work, as well as keeping you fully engaged.

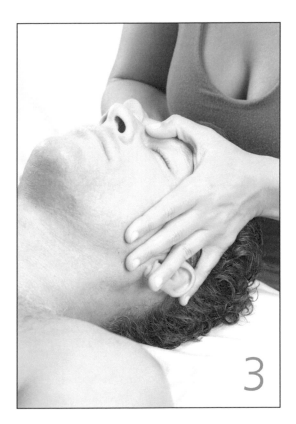

3 Trace the forehead from its center and move toward the temples. Repeat this delicate stroke, feeling the contour of the bones. Let your fingertips sink into the temples, making slow circles using firm but light pressure.

4 Trace the sides of the nose and cheekbones, moving your fingers from the undersides of the cheekbones toward the ears.

5 Take each earlobe between your thumb and forefinger and rub the ear gently from the earlobe up the sides and the tip of the ear.

6 Trace the upper lip, moving toward the jawbone.

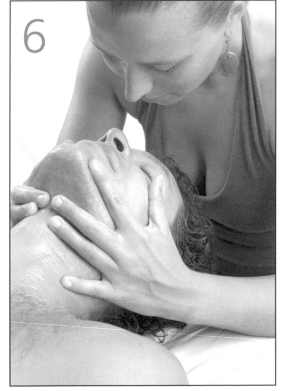

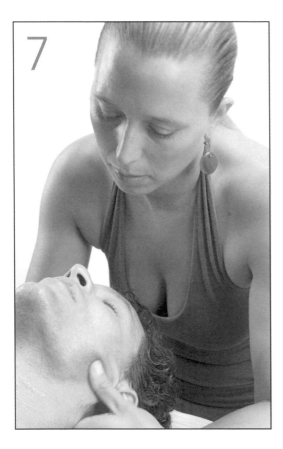

7 When you reach the joint where the jaw meets the cheekbone, make little circles in the joint of the jaw. If your partner's jaw is tight or clenched, encourage him to relax it by working the area and suggesting he open his mouth just a little so he can feel the difference. If you sense tension here, check with your partner to make sure it is not being caused by something you're doing.

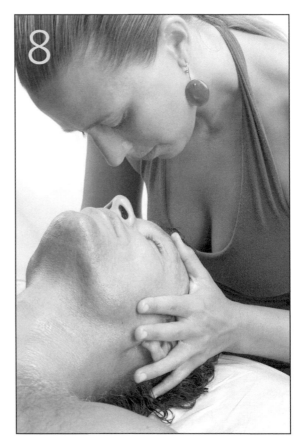

8 Use your thumb and fingers to trace the bottom and top of the jawbone. Follow the bone from the chin toward the ears in a soft lifting motion. Repeat this with an open hand, slowly caressing your partner's face with your open hands.

integrating the neck & head

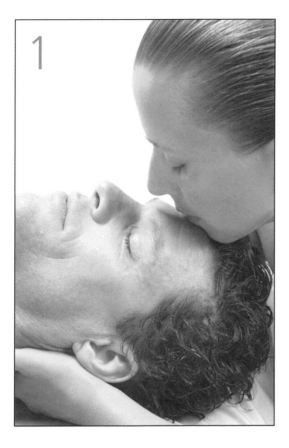

1 Come back to the head and work the scalp again. You are reinforcing the earlier work done here, and you may notice a difference in the level of relaxation your partner is experiencing now.

2 Lift the head and elongate the neck one more time, as if to say goodbye to it for the moment.

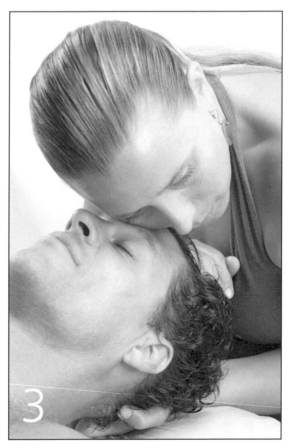

3 Bring the head back down to rest on the table and do one long stroke down the front of the body to integrate all that you have done so far.

a long stroke under the upper body

This long stroke is done with your hands under the body, while in contact with the muscles on either side of the spine. It is effective in that you can give a wonderful stretch to the receiver's body and at the same time use his body weight to apply pressure to the muscles on either side of the spine. These muscles, when tight, can contribute to pulling the vertebrae out of alignment.

This is not an easy move to do, and you should not attempt it if the receiver is bigger than you are. It is possible to injure yourself by putting too much weight on your wrists or fingers, and unless you drop your center of gravity, your back can also be compromised. Having said that, you can try a variation on this move where you slide your hands under the upper back just a little way, so as not to strain yourself. Follow the instructions below if you want to try it. If it's done well, the receiver will love it.

1 Oil up your hands and forearms.

2 Take a low, wide position with one leg ahead of the other.

3 Hold the neck with one hand, and with your other hand, palm facing upward, press the tabletop down, as you slide your hand and forearm in under the body, reaching as far as you can comfortably go. Your hand should be right under the big muscle group lateral to the spine, not on the spine itself.

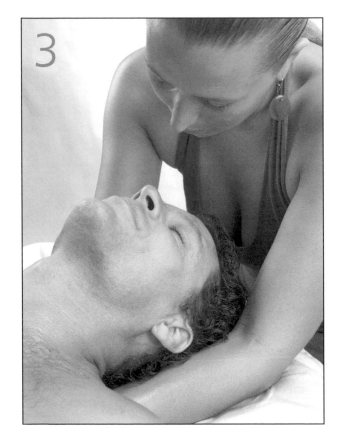

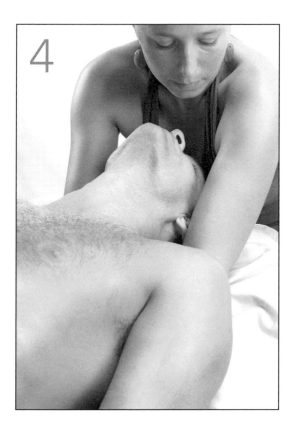

4 Now release the neck and slide your other hand under the back.

5 Adjust your palms so you are in contact with the center of the muscle group, and curl your fingers slightly.

6 Keep your center of gravity low as you lean back. Press your fingers into the muscles and pull slowly up the back. The trick is to stay low so your legs, rather than your back, do the work. Pay attention to your wrists and let up the pressure if you feel a strain. You can also do this move with your fingers flat, using your palms to press.

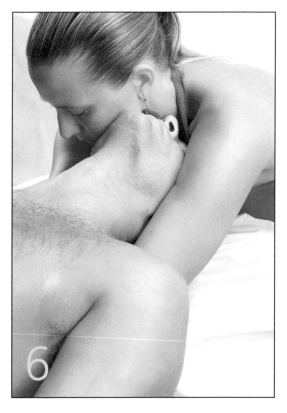

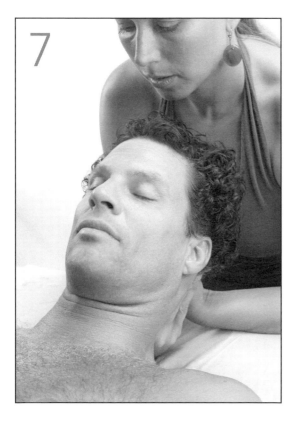

7 Complete the move by following the muscles all the way up the neck to the head, lifting it gently as you gracefully slide off the back of the head.

This is meant to be a long, smooth move, and it will take some practice to feel comfortable doing it. I suggest you repeat it a few times, trying it different ways. If your partner is heavy, you may only be able to move down the back a little way. In that case, go only as far as is comfortable and keep your hand flat on the return, rather than strain your own body. If your partner is light, you can play with this move, letting your fingers actually lift the back and elongate the spine as you move from the pelvic bone all the way up the back. At this point, another long stroke down the front of the body will integrate the work you've done. After completion, move to the side of the table and prepare to work on your partner's belly.

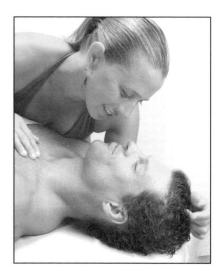

The Belly

Considering the discussion earlier regarding the front of the body, it's important to approach the belly slowly and respectfully. You'll need to pay attention to your partner's breath. Before beginning, make sure he is ready and not holding his breath. If his breath is shallow, encourage awareness by asking him to breathe deeply into his belly. Working slowly here supports trust. If you notice any changes in your partner's breath while working here, stop and check in to make sure he is comfortable with what is happening.

1 Stand at the side of the table and oil your hands.

2 On your partner's inhalation, allow the belly to rise up and meet your palms. Follow the breath as you make firm but gentle contact.

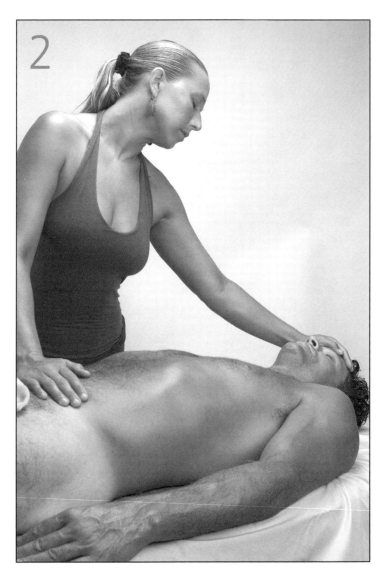

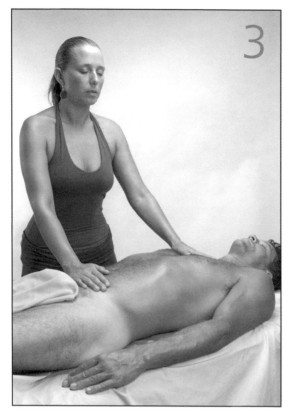

3 With your hands on the belly, ride the breath for a moment or two.

4 Begin to move your hands in a circular motion around the belly on the muscles between the ribs and the pubic bone. One hand follows the other moving in a clockwise motion to support the path of digestion.

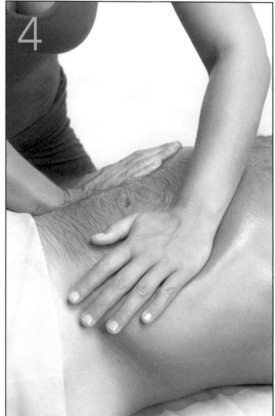

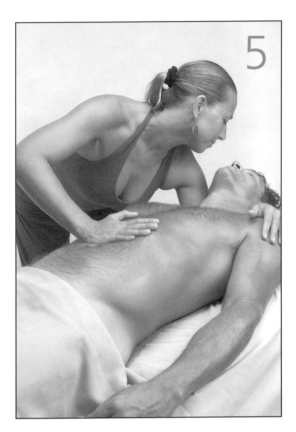

5 Now slide one hand under the lower back to provide support as the other hand continues making slow circles on the belly. The hand that rests on the back gives support to the area both physically and emotionally. It's like the mother hand, always there support-ing, not always doing or moving.

6 Take a wide stance facing the table. Bring both hands to the belly. Now bring the hand closest to the head slowly up the chest, around the shoulder, way under the neck, to the opposite shoulder to cradle the neck in your arm and hand. Take a breath here and enjoy the intimacy of the moment. Your partner will feel secure and nur-tured by this support.

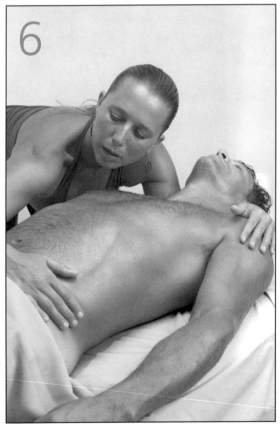

7 The hand resting on the belly now begins to make circles again—small ones along the muscles, larger ones across the whole area between the ribs and hips. Work in this way for a few minutes, or as long as is comfortable for you both.

8 To transition from this move, let the hand that was circling ride softly up the midline of the chest to the top of the sternum and meet the hand that has been supporting the neck. Then come down the arm and off the fingertips.

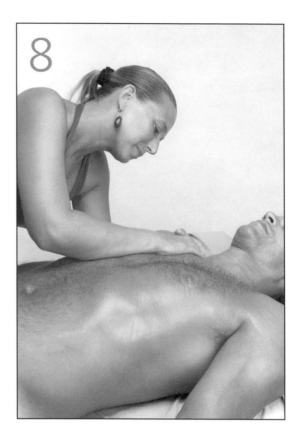

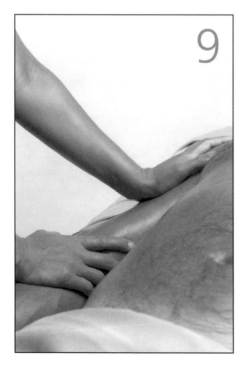

9 Give a little traction or pull of the arm at the shoulder before continuing down the arm to the hands and off the fingertips. End slowly. Any rushing at the end of the move negates what went before it, leaving the receiver confused and not relaxed.

The last stroke connects the work done on the belly with the upper chest, shoulder, arms, and hands, and is a transition move to the next place you will massage: the arms and hands.

The Hands

When working on the extremities, you are more distant from the core of your partner's body, but the work can be just as intimate. Take your time to explore the bones of the hands and arms. Enjoy moving each finger and rotating the wrists.

1 Oil your hands in preparation for massaging the arms and hands. Lift your partner's hand and hold it between both of yours for a moment. What feeling can you convey simply in the hand hold?

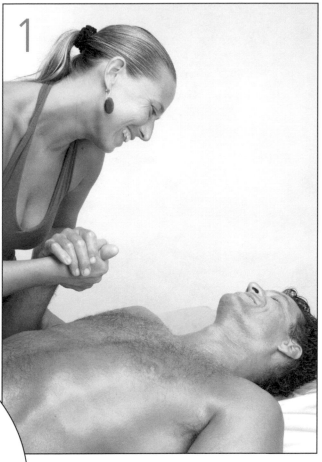

2 Let your love flow between your palms as you refocus your intention to your partner's hand. Begin to rub the top of the hand with your palms.

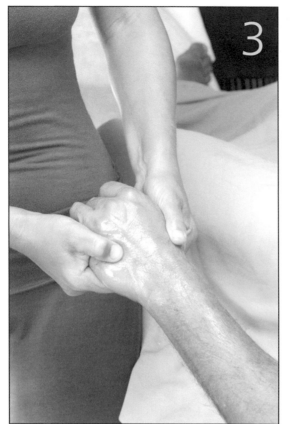

3 Using your fingers, trace the valleys between the tendons on the tops of the hands.

4 Pull each finger as you massage them on all sides. Gently squeeze the nail as you leave the finger.

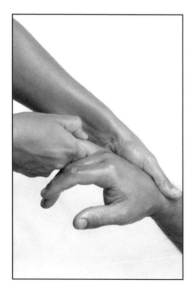

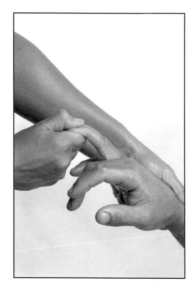

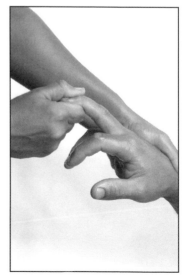

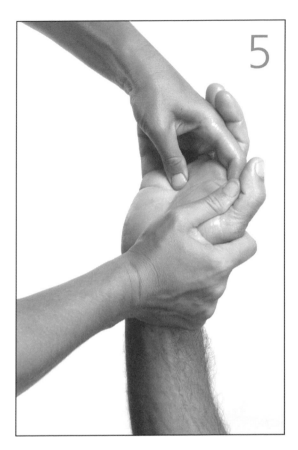

5 Turn the hand over so the palm faces you. Use your thumbs to massage the palm by spreading the bones and opening the hand. Explore the movement of the bones.

6 Include the wrist in your hand massage. Interlace your fingers and rotate the hand and wrist in both directions.

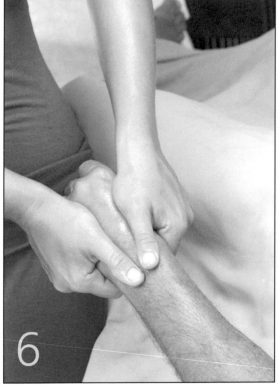

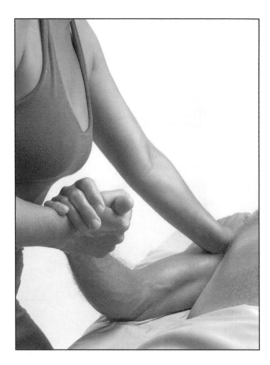

The Arms

When lifting the arm, always support the elbow joint. If stretching the arm overhead, bring the hand up the midline of the body so as not to compress the shoulder joint. If your partner feels supported, it will be easy for him to give up holding tension. Remember to work in a meaningful way and move slowly when working on the extremities.

1 Continue to hold the wrist with one hand so as to anchor the arm and not jam it into the shoulder when working up the arm. Oil the arm.

2 Gently knead the muscles of the upper arm and then the muscles between the bones of the forearm, all the way back to the wrist and hand.

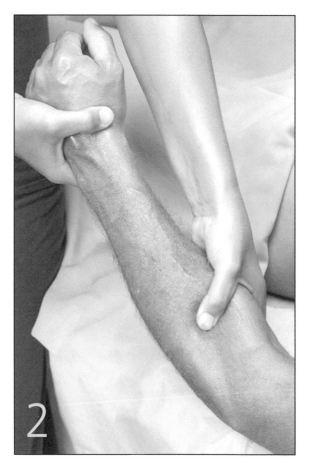

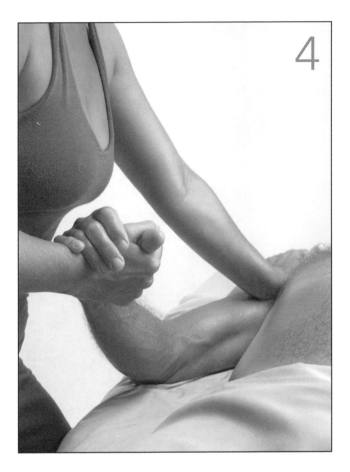

3 Hold your partner's wrist with his arm bent at a forty-five degree angle. Swing it gently back and forth, releasing any tension in the joint.

4 Lovingly hold your partner's hand in yours for a moment before carefully placing it back on the table or on his belly.

5 Stay there for a moment before softly breaking contact.

At this point, you will go to the opposite side of the table and balance the work you did on the first side by repeating it on the other side. It is not necessary to keep a hand on the body as you move from place to place. Allow space for both of you to integrate, and when you are touching, be fully there and not moving around or reaching for your oil.

When you are ready to begin and reconnect, do so slowly and gently. Experience the melding of your hand and your partner's belly. Repeat the circling moves, still working in a clockwise direction, and repeat the cradling on this side of the body as well. As you complete the belly work, bring your stoke up the front of the arm to the wrist. Then reach across the body to the other wrist and gently pull them equally, so as not to leave the body lopsided. At this point, some people will take a spontaneous deep breath indicating release. Massage your partner's other arm and hand.

integrating the front of the body

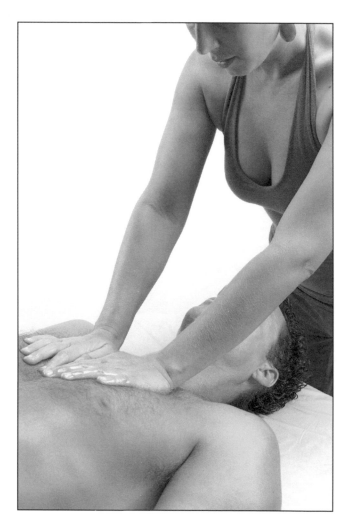

You can now integrate all the work you have done on the front of the body by doing another long, slow stroke starting at the chest and moving down the front, back up, and around the shoulders, finishing at the neck and head. Carefully place the head back on the table and remain in contact briefly before coming away.

This is a good time for the giver to stretch and drink some water, before quietly returning to the foot of the table to work on the feet and legs. The receiver may need to stretch or drink a glass of water too, or just to move around or make some adjustments to his comfort. It's also a good time to check in with your partner and see how he's doing. When you're both ready, you can begin by standing or sitting on a stool at the foot of the table.

The Feet

For most people, there is no such thing as too much work on the feet. So even though you have done some work on the other side of the foot, it's important to do focused work from this side as well, since you can access different areas. Imagine how much work your feet do and how much weight they carry. It's easy to love your beloved's feet as his foundation, his support, and his transport. Give them all the time and energy they need. It's a good place to lose yourself, simply feeling the work from a loving place, without regard to technique. Here are some guidelines to follow. Use oil as necessary.

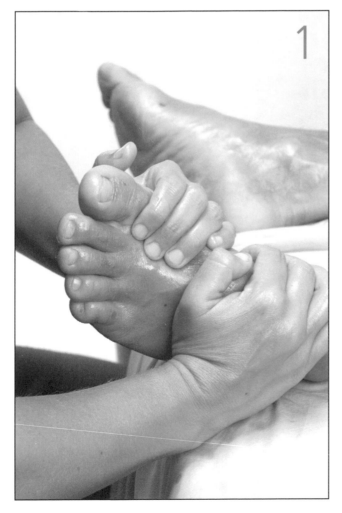

1 Massage the tops of the feet with your palms as well as your fingers. Gently squeeze the tissue in your hands.

2 Run your fingers and thumbs between the tendons on the tops of the feet.

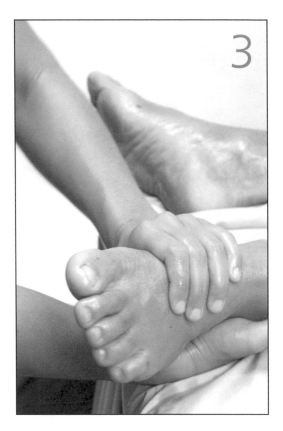

3 Press on the ball of the foot with your palms or thumbs to spread the bones and tissue.

4 Press all around the heel and stretch the instep by flexing the foot.

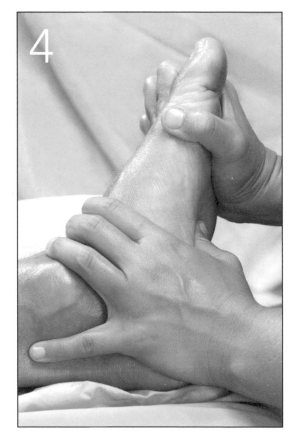

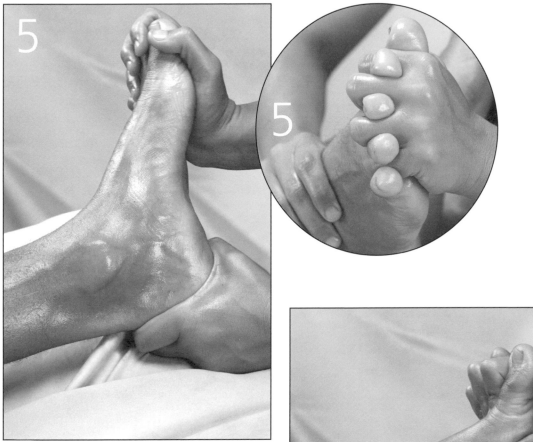

5 Hold the heel in your palms and interlace your fingers between the toes. Support the heel and rotate the ankle in both directions.

6 Lean slightly into your hands as you press against the foot. This causes the bones to spread and the foot to feel wider and more open.

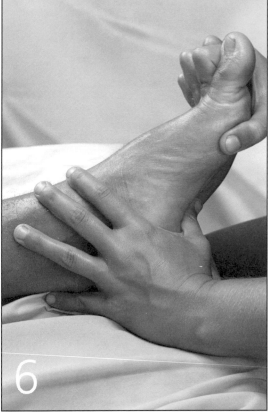

7 Massage each toe, one at a time, and trace the valleys between the toes.

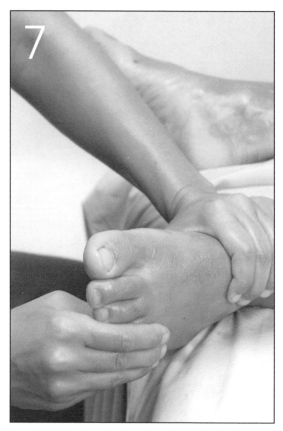

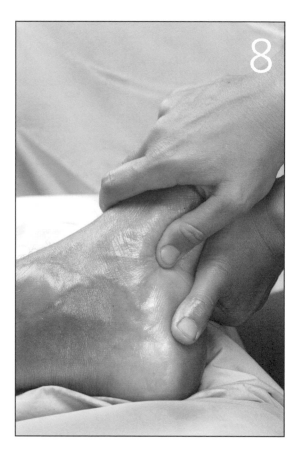

8 Now just enjoy massaging your partner's foot and do what comes naturally. Close your eyes and lovingly massage his foot, caressing, squeezing, spreading, and stretching it. Trust your intuition.

9 Close your foot massage in a sweet way and move to the other foot.

10 Repeat the same work you just did on the first foot.

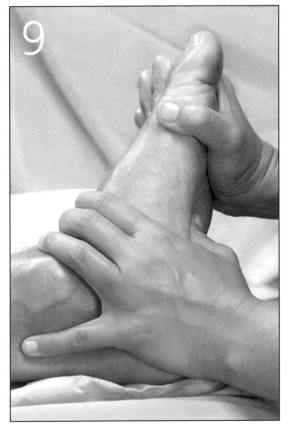

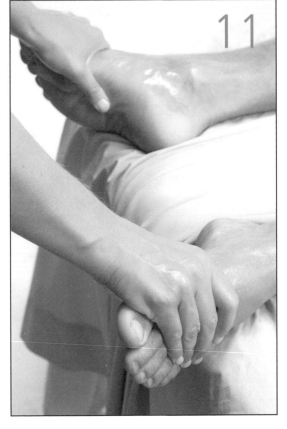

11 When both feet have been well massaged, let your hands rest on the tops of both of them in a quiet hold. You are now ready to move from the feet to the legs.

connecting the legs & upper body

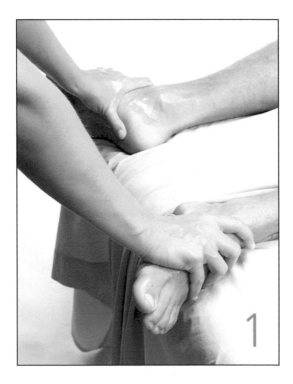

1 Apply some oil to your hands and stand at the foot of the table.

2 Connect on the top of your partner's foot, before doing a long stroke up the front of the leg to the hip, and back down to the foot. If you can't make the long reach to the hip, go to the side of the table, where you are free to move and don't have to stretch.

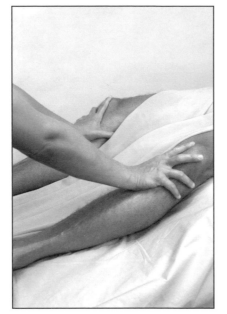

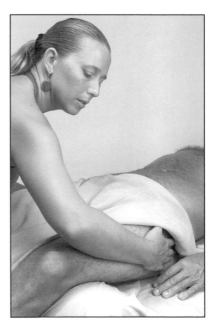

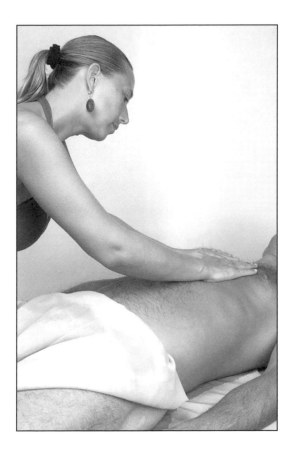

3 Once the leg has been oiled, you will do a long stroke from the foot, up the leg and belly and chest, along the collarbone to the shoulder, and down the arm to the hand and fingertips. This smooth stroke connects the lower and upper body on one side, and helps the receiver integrate the work.

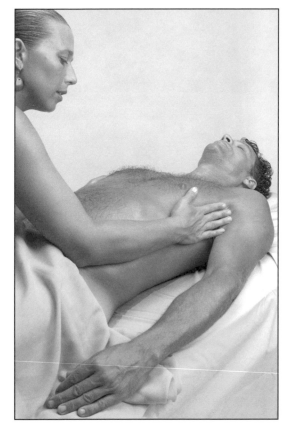

4 Now you can do the same move using both hands together on either side of the body. Start at the side of the table and move along the table, touching your partner with firm, gentle contact from his toes to his fingertips. Use your body-weight to lean into this move, and it will begin to feel like dance. For the receiver, it might feel like one long breath.

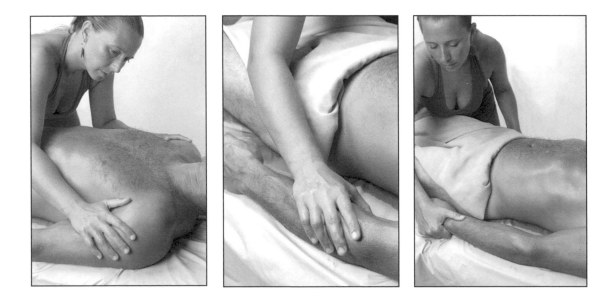

5 Repeat this long slow stroke two or three times on each side to get more comfortable doing it.

Your partner's body will feel integrated, and you can now bring your attention to the leg.

The Legs

1 Begin standing and facing your partner's leg. Place one hand on his hip and the other on his foot.

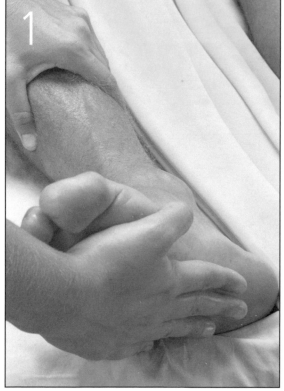

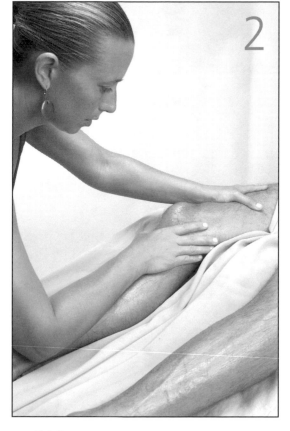

2 Gently rock the leg toward the midline of the body and allow it to fall back to its natural resting place. Rhythmic gentle rocking of the leg will help relax tension in the hip.

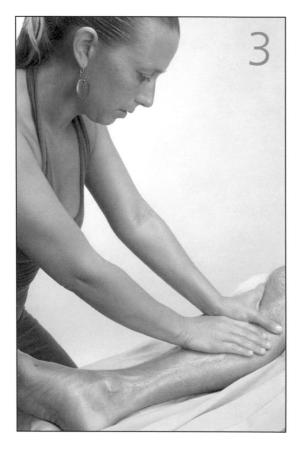

3 Now oil your hands and prepare to do another long stroke up the leg. This time, lean into your hands by bending your knees, keeping your back and arms straight, and moving from your center.

 Work gently around the knee.

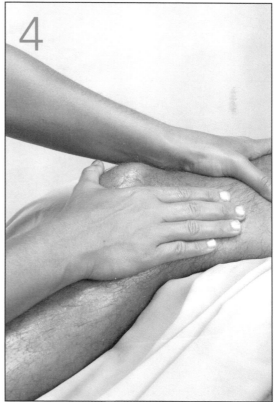

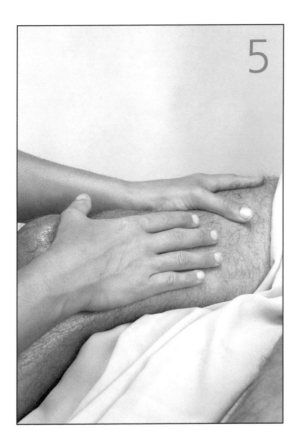

5 When you reach the thigh, where there is a bigger muscle mass, apply more pressure with more weight and spread your hands wide.

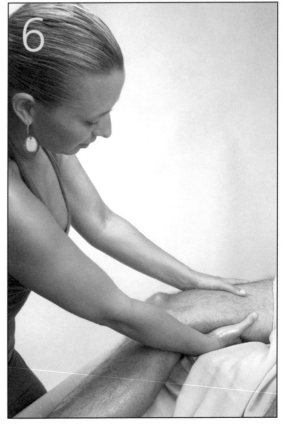

6 Come around the hip bone, and with one hand on the top of the leg and one hand under it, shift your weight to your back leg as you come down the leg and return to the foot. This three-dimensional move gives your partner a feeling of connectedness as well as movement, since by lightly pulling on the leg you are also effecting movement of the spine.

7 Repeat the above moves at least twice before moving to the side of the table to knead the calf muscles and work your way to the thigh muscles.

8 Massage along the grain of the thigh muscle as well as across the grain of the muscle. Use your fingers as well as your palms, and try alternating your hands as they move from the knee to the hip bone.

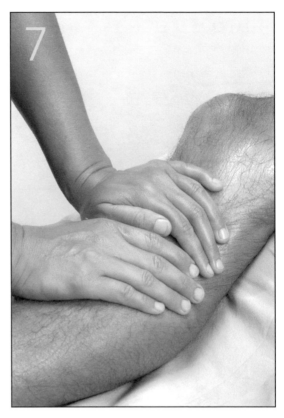

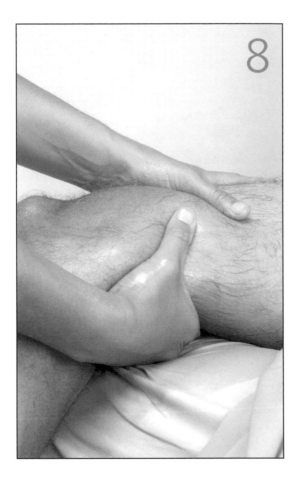

9 Return to the foot and get ready for the hip stretch.

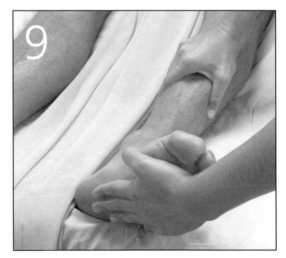

hip stretch

This is a gentle stretch, and if you work together, it should be easy and comfortable for you both. Be sure to stay connected, giving feedback as necessary. The purpose of this move is to explore the range of motion in the hip and elongate the tightened muscles.

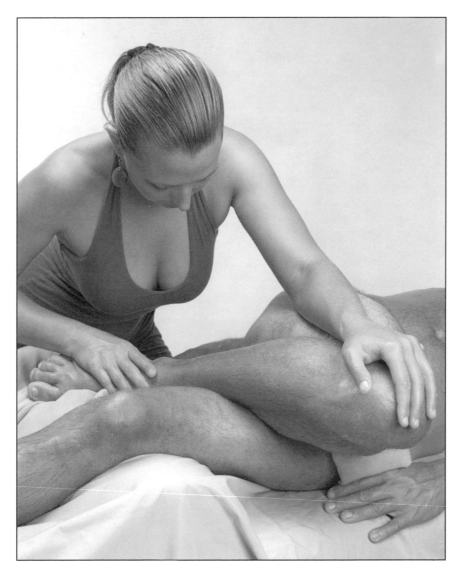

1 Stand at the side of the table facing your partner's legs.

2 Gently lift the leg nearest you, bending the knee. Place the foot flat on the table next to the other knee, so the bent leg is at a ninety-degree angle to the other one.

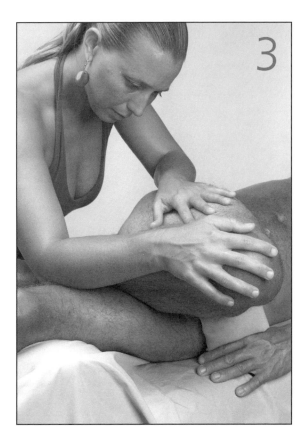

3 Now, with one hand on the knee and one hand firmly on the hip, slowly roll your partner's leg away from you, stretching both his hip and leg muscles. Go very slowly and pay attention to your partner's breath. Lean into the leg for a further stretch, and work with the breath by giving pressure on an exhalation. Stay within your partner's range of comfort.

4 When you've come to the limit of the stretch, support the knee and foot and return the leg to the table.

5 Another long stroke completes and integrates the work on this leg.

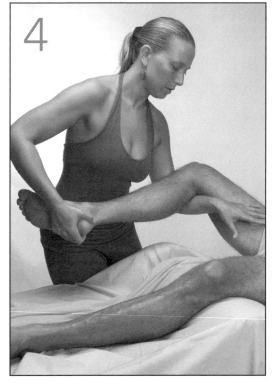

Move to the other leg and repeat all the moves. Since most people are not perfectly balanced, you may find that one side stretches more easily than the other. When you have completed both legs, you will connect the entire body again with a long, sensuous stroke from toes to fingertips. You can repeat this several times and vary your timing and pressure, moving more slowly and delicately each time.

completing the massage

Come back to the head of the table and find your own way to complete the massage or say goodbye. This can be anything from stillness to repeated moves, from sensual touch to extremely light contact. Take the time to finish in a way that is personal to you. When these final strokes are done, move to the side of the table. Place one hand on the crown of your partner's head and the other on your partner's center or belly. Close your eyes, connecting to your own breath first and then to each other. Feel the energy flow between you. Honor and give thanks for each other and for the shared blessing of what you've experienced together.

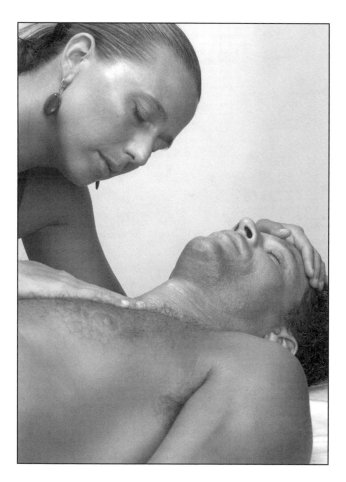

Take as much time as you need before separating, and do so quietly and slowly. When you do, give each other plenty of time before breaking the feeling of the moment with words. The receiver has had an inward journey and needs time to return. The giver has been putting her energy out and may need a moment before connecting again. Now is a good time for the giver to wash your hands and shake them out.

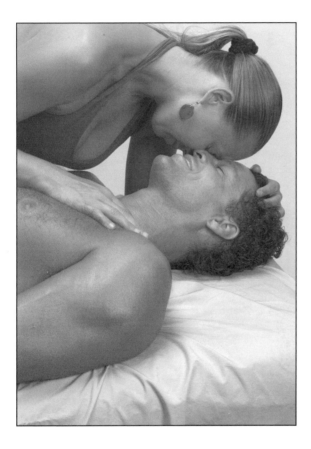

Stretch and breathe and take some time for yourself, while your partner slowly returns. You may feel so moved that words are inappropriate, so sharing can come later on. Stay with your experience as long as possible, and when the time is right, share it with each other. Offer your partner water and make sure he is warm enough. Enjoy the connection you've just experienced, and allow the sweetness of the moment to encompass you both.

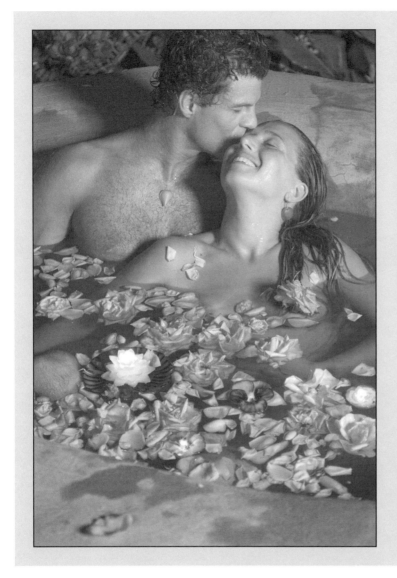

ENDING WITH A BATH

After the massage, share a bath filled with your favorite fragrance, flowers, and floating candles or bubbles. Relax together and luxuriate in its soothing water. Share this precious time together and make it a commitment to do so more often.

CHAPTER 3

THE BACKRUB & THE NECK & SHOULDER MASSAGE

In this chapter, I'll teach the backrub and the neck and shoulder massage, each a different and wonderful way to connect and share with each other. The backrub is given in a leisurely way, so more intimacy can follow. The neck and shoulder massage can be done with the receiver clothed and seated or standing anywhere. It can be short or take fifteen minutes or more. Almost any amount of loving touch will be well received by you both, and it is good to practice your skills at both these ways of nurturing each other.

THE BACKRUB

Is there a person alive who doesn't love a backrub? Maybe someone who has never received one would fall into that category, but for many couples a backrub is a delicious treat shared on a regular basis. It not only feels really good, it can be therapeutic by helping each of you release the tension and pain from your body. Learning how to work together in this way furthers your connection, your communication, and your compassion for each other as much as it nourishes the relationship. You don't even need a table to give and receive a backrub. The floor, covered with a mat, or the bed will do fine. It can be offered on special occasions or on a lazy afternoon of lovemaking. Anytime is a good time for a backrub.

PREPARATION

Whatever the occasion, you'll want to take a couple of moments to prepare yourselves and the space.

The Space

Create some quiet space, just as you would do in a full body massage. It is important to massage each other when you are both relaxed and receptive, at the end of the day or in the evening. Create your time and intimate space together.

Light a candle, use an aromatic lotion or oil, and put on some soft music. Unplug your phone. Let time slip away.

Learn what makes each other purr and give each other the gift of a beautiful backrub.

Setting the Intention of the Backrub

Together you will set the intention of the backrub. First, communicate about what each of you needs. Ask each other where you experience the tension. Ask each other what would feel really good. Share with each other the places that hurt or feel vulnerable. Ask for what you want.

The amount of time you spend is completely up to you. You can do great work in just a few moments or enjoy the luxury of a nice long backrub if time allows. It can be as sensual as you allow, as well as healing and therapeutic. For some couples, the backrub is a prelude to lovemaking, a beautiful way to begin. It can also be just a backrub, delicious and complete in itself. The exchange makes it win for both of you, so be generous in giving and receiving. It will bring you closer, and your appreciation for each other will grow as you learn to help relieve each other's pain as well as give each other pleasure.

The Receiver's Position

If you're the receiver, make yourself comfortable on the bed or a mat on the floor. Lie facedown, with your head turned to one side. Remember to occasionally turn your head from one side to the other so your neck doesn't get stiff. If there is discomfort in your neck, bring your arm up next to your head to relieve some of the pressure on the neck and shoulder. Your feet can hang off the end of the bed. If you're using a mat on the floor, insert a pillow under your ankles for support. Your arms can be at your side or above your head, whichever feels better. A pillow placed under your hips helps relieve discomfort due to lower back compression. Use as many pillows as it takes to get comfortable. If you're on the floor, you may need an extra cover or more heat. Make sure you're comfortable before beginning.

The Giver's Position

The best position I've found for giving a backrub is to straddle the receiver's body at the hips. This works for my husband and me because our weight does not greatly differ. If you are a lot bigger than the receiver, you will have to support your own weight, rather than sitting on your partner's buttocks.

Start by kneeling while straddling the back, and slowly let your weight transfer from your legs as you sit gingerly on your partner's buttocks, testing the application of your weight before settling into a comfortable position for you both. You may need to place pillows behind your knees for support and comfort. You will be shifting your weight from a sitting position to your knees and back again.

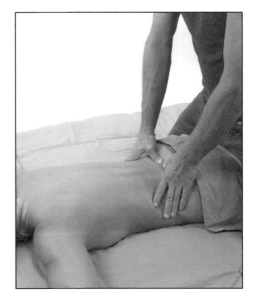

Another way to approach the backrub is by kneeling at your partner's head. You will still be shifting your weight and kneeling, but there is no pressure on your partner's body from your own weight. Find the most comfortable position for you both, and use whatever support you need, such as pillows behind your knees or a blanket to kneel on.

The Back

The intention of the work on the back is to open it by elongating the spine, smoothing the tired muscles that hold us erect, applying traction to the sacrum and lower back, and creating more space between the ribs to facilitate deeper breathing. You must always begin slowly and gently, and let your partner relax and open at her own speed. Make the transition into bliss slow and sensual, and enjoy each move. Let the first strokes be firm and gentle, introducing your touch. As you spread the oil, you can feel the muscles of the back and determine how to best support your partner with your healing touch.

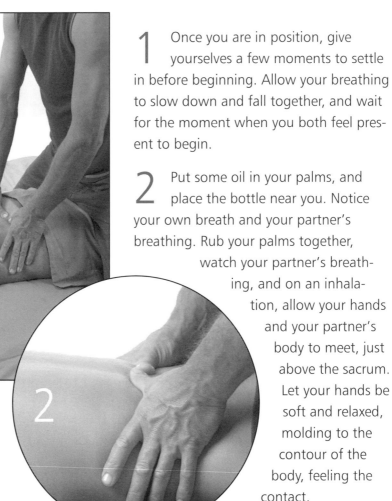

1 Once you are in position, give yourselves a few moments to settle in before beginning. Allow your breathing to slow down and fall together, and wait for the moment when you both feel present to begin.

2 Put some oil in your palms, and place the bottle near you. Notice your own breath and your partner's breathing. Rub your palms together, watch your partner's breathing, and on an inhalation, allow your hands and your partner's body to meet, just above the sacrum. Let your hands be soft and relaxed, molding to the contour of the body, feeling the contact.

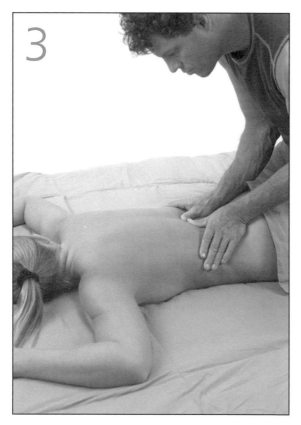

3 Wait for another exhalation, and then begin a long, slow stroke up the back. As you approach the mid back, begin shifting your weight forward. As you come to your knees, move your weight into your hands and apply more pressure to the mid back as your partner exhales. Continue your stroke along the shoulders to the arms and give the muscles of the arms a little squeeze. Then travel back down to the hands, pausing a moment before leaving at the fingertips.

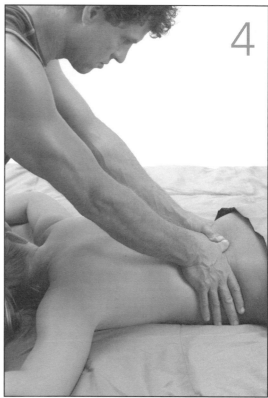

4 Repeat this long, slow move several times, as you spread the oil on your partner's back and get a feeling for where the tension is. Alternate your hands to create rhythm and change. Keep your weight behind your hands as you lovingly move along the muscles on either side of the spine, giving your body weight to your hands.

5 After you have oiled your partner's back with enough oil or lotion so your moves can be smooth, set your oil aside.

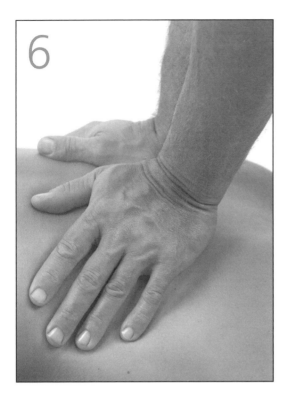

6 Begin softly, using light strokes at first to get your partner relaxed and used to your touch.

7 You can vary your long strokes by changing your weight and by using your arms, wrists, and forearms to relieve the pressure on your wrists and hands. They are broader tools, and you can apply more pressure when using them. Work slowly, with awareness of breath. Wait for an exhalation to apply more pressure. It becomes easier to give strong pressure once you've learned how to use your body weight.

8 On your partner's exhalation, increase your pressure gradually, and be ready to respond to feedback.

Keep your conversation to a minimum, and let your exchange be about what is happening in the moment. A simple sigh or sound will indicate appreciation or discomfort. Let each other know what feels good and what you want.

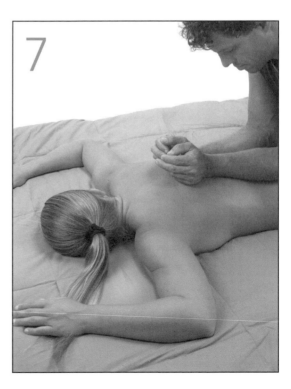

The Neck, Shoulders, Spine, & Ribs

1 Now move up the back to the shoulders. Use your palms to massage the shoulder muscles, working them from their contracted, forward position toward a softened, relaxed one. Try squeezing them lightly and see if your partner likes it. For some it feels wonderful, and others don't care for it. Find out what he likes on the shoulders. Some people like direct pressure right on the muscle, while others prefer more general

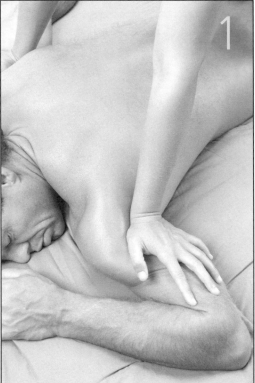

work in the area instead. Continue from the shoulders into the neck. Work on the side that is available, and then ask you partner to turn his head the other way so you can work on that side as well.

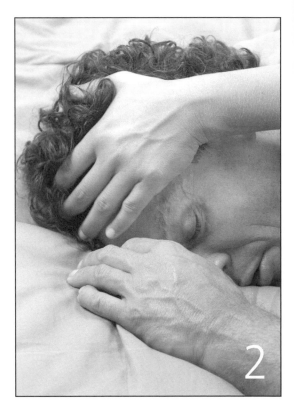

2 Work into the hairline and the head and scalp, massaging with your fingertips.

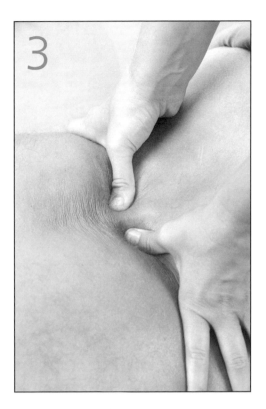

3 Now, with your fingertips on either side of the spine, explore the shape and mobility of your partner's spine. Gently move your fingertips along each vertebra, from the base of the spine to the top of the neck.

4 Bring your palms to the shoulders and lightly knead the shoulder muscles. This area can be very sensitive and tight, as people tend to "shoulder" life's worries or fears there. Approach your partner with sensitivity, and never work too fast or too deep. Check with your partner regarding pressure. Think about encouraging the

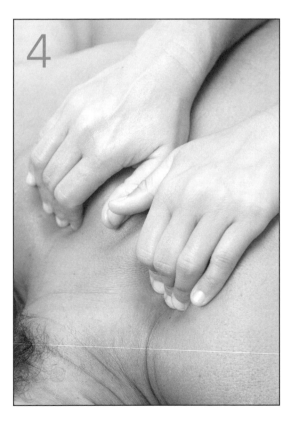

shoulders from their tightened, forward position back to a natural, relaxed one. Knead the muscles using your fingers or palms, adding a little squeeze if your partner is comfortable with that. Include the muscles of the neck, and massage them from the base of the neck to the hairline. Massaging the head can be wonderfully relaxing and sensual, so take your time and give your partner's head some attention. Massage the scalp and move it across the bones of the skull. Lightly pull your partner's hair. Sensually comb your partner's hair with your fingers.

5 Place your hands in the prayer position, and using the edge of your hands as your tool, apply increasing pressure to the mid back area, where there can be a lot of tension. Be sure your partner is comfortable with this move and that the pressure is not too much for her. Between moves, ask your partner to move her head from side to side slowly, with a rest in the middle before turning fully. This will relieve stress on the neck. Ask her to take a deep breath and exhale as you increase your weight.

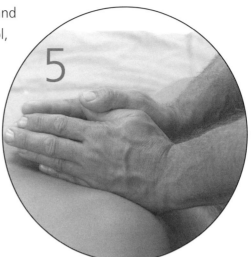

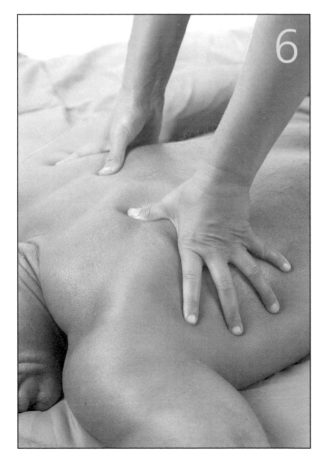

6 Work along the ribs of the back, first defining them and lightly massaging the muscles between the ribs. This work encourages deeper breath and helps brings the receiver's awareness to his breathing. If ticklishness is an issue, try using more rather than less pressure or avoid those areas completely. Suggest that the receiver try focusing on his breath if he feels ticklish. This usually works. Alternate your stroke on the ribs, working along them and then across them. Let your hands dance over your partner's body.

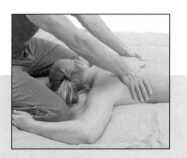

ALTERNATE POSITION FOR THE GIVER

Working from the head of the body, the moves are reversed. You will start by connecting on the upper back and moving down to the hips, up the ribs, along the arms, and off the fingertips or off the top of the head. You can increase your weight as you begin to move down the back and let up at the lumbar spine, where there are no ribs to provide support. Never put direct, heavy pressure on the spine itself. Work the hips by making little circles between the bones of the pelvis and hips, pressing deeply into the body for more pressure. Trace the deeper muscles with your palms, working slowly.

7 If you are straddling your partner's back, gradually let your weight down onto your partner's hips. By weighting your partner's hips, you are giving them traction and inviting the lower back to open and elongate. If there are problems in the lower back, this traction can feel very good. Again, be sensitive and slow in applying your weight, and if your partner feels uncomfortable, don't do it. You can work on the sacrum, the V-shaped bone at the end of the spine. Trace it with your fingers and find the *sacroiliac joint,* where there are often two dimples. If more weight is desired, get up on your knees, weight your hands on the sacrum, and pull back toward yourself as you move down the sacrum and into the muscles of the hips, lightening your stroke and letting the pressure off easily.

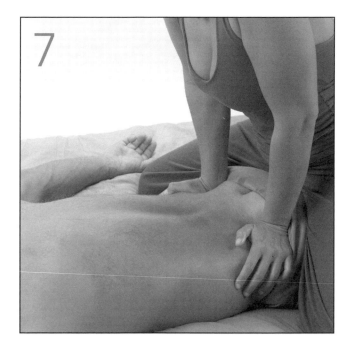

cross strokes & compression moves

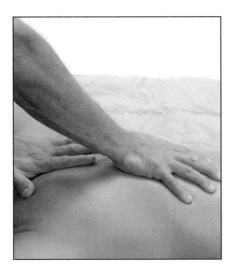

Cross strokes give a nice variation here and allow you to contact the ribs and the side of the body. You can move to the side of your partner's body and work across the ribs, waist, and hips, one hand following the other in slow, rhythmic motion as you move up and down the torso. Repeat all your moves on the other side of the body as well.

Compression moves are also very effective and feel good to the receiver. In these moves, the giver puts direct pressure or compression on an area of the body. They are used where there is more body mass, such as the back and thighs. The weight is always applied on an exhalation. Compression moves can be done from the side of the body or from either end.

With your shoulders directly over your palms, begin to move your weight into your hands. Go slowly, applying more weight a little at a time. Work with your partner's breathing so as he is exhaling, you are putting the weight in your hands. Encourage sound on the exhalation, particularly if you are going deep and adding a lot of weight.

Work with each other closely, and be sure to respond to your partner's request for more or less pressure. Don't assume you know what's right for each other. "No pain, no gain" is also not true. The body resists pain, and too much pressure can cause a fight-or-flight response, making the muscles tighter rather than softer. There is a fine line between pleasure and pain, and it's important to stay in your partner's comfort zone. That way you are working together, and there is little resistance. Your loving presence with each other is what encourages trust, relaxation, and letting go.

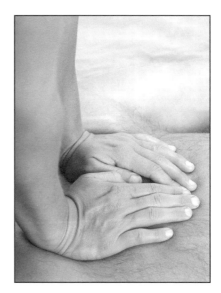

completing the backrub

Repeat the long stoke from the hips up the back, down the arms, and off the fingers. This reconnects the parts of the back you have worked on separately. Repeat this move several times, varying it by using your fingers, hands, and forearms. Change your rhythm, and repeat strokes that feel good. Respond to the *oohs* and *aahs* of your partner by continuing a move she especially likes. Make up strokes and use props to make it more fun. Try using a feather, or a piece of silk, or your fingernails, or your own long hair for a sensual stroke down the back. Make your backrub sensual and fun. Sometimes it will lead to a wonderful evening of lovemaking. It is a perfect way to relax and get in tune with each other. You'll probably want to trade backrubs first!

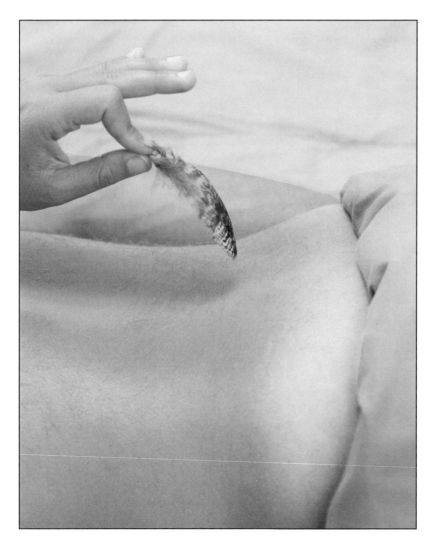

THE BACKRUB USING SUPPORT

For great results and minimum effort, my husband and I often use a hassock as support in doing a great backrub. My husband likes to kneel on the floor and lie facedown over the hassock. I can exert a lot of pressure by leveraging my body weight in this position, as he allows the form to support his back in this wide-open position. I straddle the bolster and work along his back this way, or stand or kneel facing his back at the head. Either way, I can get a lot of pressure in my hands by leaning directly into them. If I am kneeling, my forearms are the best tool, and standing, I use my hands more. This type of work is more about compression and pressure than about long soothing strokes, although it is always good to add a few. It can be incredibly therapeutic in a short time.

Depending on your body, and what is available to you and comfortable for you, this exact position may or may not work. You may find something in your own home to perfectly support your body.

For the receiver, just the act of stretching your torso out over the hassock is opening in itself. The ribs expand and there is space for the spine to elongate, without the pull of gravity.

The giver can straddle the bolster over your partner's hips and remain standing, unless you are light enough to gently sit just below the sacrum.

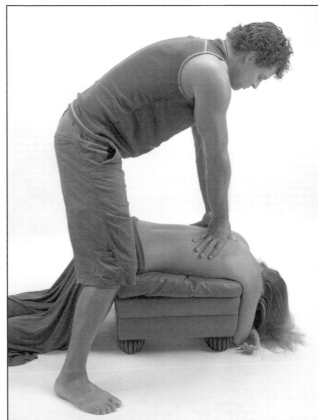

The Back

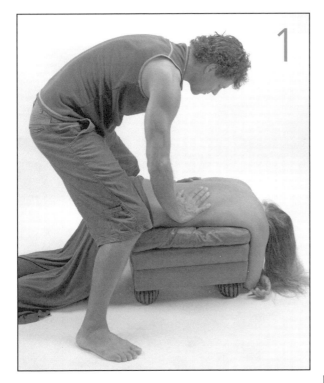

1 Begin with a long stroke up the back to the shoulder, and return. Cover the back with lotion so your hands glide easily over the skin. The main muscle groups you are working on are along either side of the spine. They become tight from holding us erect, and from the work they do as we lift things and move through life. Tension is carried in the back and the shoulders, and those muscles love to be coaxed to release that tension. You can soften them first with some long strokes, gradually adding more weight to your work.

2 Begin to apply more pressure by putting your weight directly over your hands and leaning on them. Be sure to work slowly and be receptive to feedback so you don't work with too much weight or pressure.

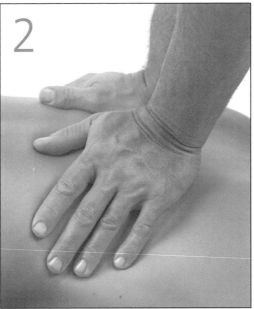

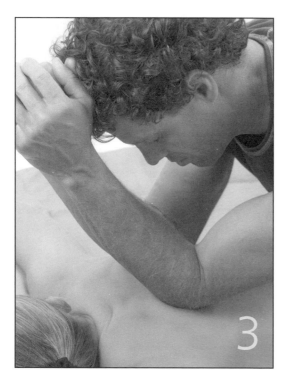

3 This is another place you can try forearms, wrists, and elbows. Always take care to go slowly, and stay off the spine itself. Continue to ask for feedback from your partner regarding pressure. Be careful not to apply too much weight, and never go too deep by ignoring her comfort zone.

4 Alternate moving your hands up the back, gradually adding your body weight. Feel yourself almost ironing out the muscles on either side of the spine, as they elongate in response to your pressure.

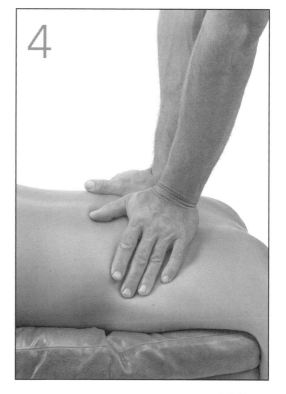

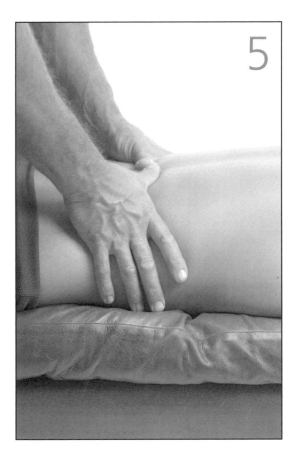

5 If you find trouble spots—places where there is a knot, or tension held in the tissue—you can use your fingers to work back and forth on the spot, your palms to rub it, or your weight to apply direct pressure to the spot. Keep a constant dialogue going regarding pressure. Your partner's breath will deepen as she lets go.

6 After you have worked deeply on a spot, always take some time to soothe it with gentle, loving strokes before transitioning to another area.

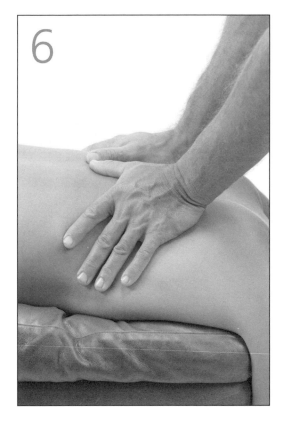

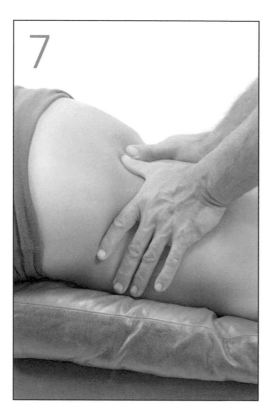

7 Work the sacrum down toward to feet, giving the lumbar spine some room to elongate and open. Using your fingertips and your palms, rub the sacrum itself and focus on the sacroiliac joints.

8 Begin a long stroke moving down the back. Cup your hands to make an open fist, with the top side in contact with the back. Begin by placing your open fists between your partner's shoulder blades.

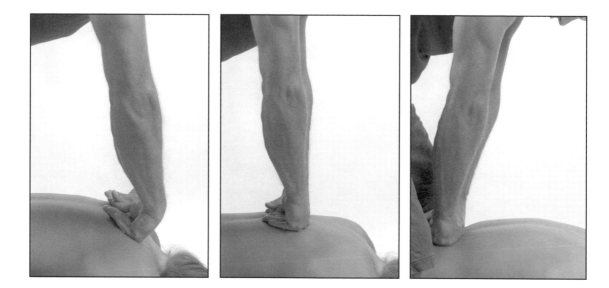

THE BACKRUB

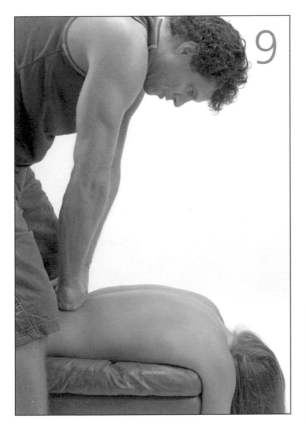

9 With your weight directly over your hands, begin to draw the muscles down the back. Move slowly, with attention to applying the right amount of pressure. Take the stroke all the way down back to the sacrum and let up there, as bone on bone is uncomfortable.

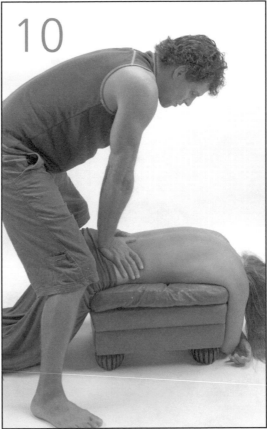

10 Turn your hands over and use your palms to massage the sacrum.

11 Complete this work with some soothing strokes down the back, then feather your fingers along the ribs and spine. Rest your hands gently on your partner's back for a moment before slowly straightening your own back and standing.

Now is the time to stretch after bending over several minutes. Elongate your spine and breathe deeply. Give your partner plenty of time to unfold and return.

AN ALTERNATIVE POSITION

If you don't have a hassock or the proper support, you can do this same work by the receiver assuming the child's pose on the floor or a mat. The *child's pose* is a resting pose in yoga, as well as a passive relaxing stretch. Your knees are bent, your belly is resting on your thighs, your arms are resting by your side and your forehead is touching the floor. Not everyone is comfortable in this position. Knee problems can make this difficult. Sometimes a pillow behind the knees can help relieve the pressure there.

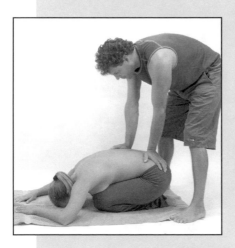

The giver can kneel facing the receiver's head and work from there. You can also straddle the back, but without placing weight on your partner's hips. If you are both comfortable in these positions, try this alternative. A session working in this way should be short, since it is difficult for both of you to maintain these postures for too long without creating discomfort. Start with five minutes and work your way up to ten, or whatever is comfortable for you. Never hurt yourselves, either giving or receiving.

Stretch and encourage your partner to take his time, moving very slowly limb by limb back to standing.

the receiver's steps to standing

The receiver should move with awareness very slowly from this position.

1 When you are ready, slide your hips back to your heels and let your arms follow with your hands touching the floor. The giver can assist here by moving the hassock out of the way.

2 You can then go to your hand and knees.

3 One foot at a time, begin to slowly stand.

4 Let your arms hang down, and come to a standing position by unfolding your spine one vertebra at a time until you are erect. Let your head follow last.

THE NECK & SHOULDER MASSAGE

Suppose your honey comes home tired and tense from a hard day. What can you do to support him, make him more comfortable? How can you listen in a way that comforts without words? Wait until he has settled in a bit, then offer a neck, head, and shoulder massage. This can be done anywhere: at a desk, at the dining room table, in an easy chair. There is no need for the receiver to remove clothes; just loosen the buttons near the neck, and let yourself be nourished. You don't need oil or lotion to do this massage. All you need is your loving intention in your hands.

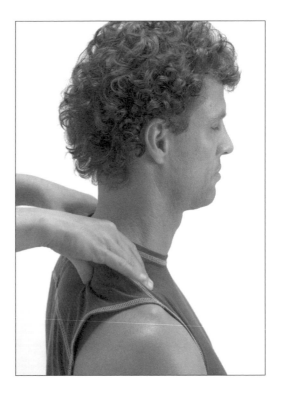

giving a neck & shoulder massage while standing

1 Stand next to your partner so you are comfortable, balanced, and relaxed and gently approach her offering your touch.

2 Connect on the shoulder, resting your palms softly on the muscles of the shoulders, and wait for breath.

3 Begin to massage the muscles through the shirt, working gently at first to determine the right pressure for your partner.

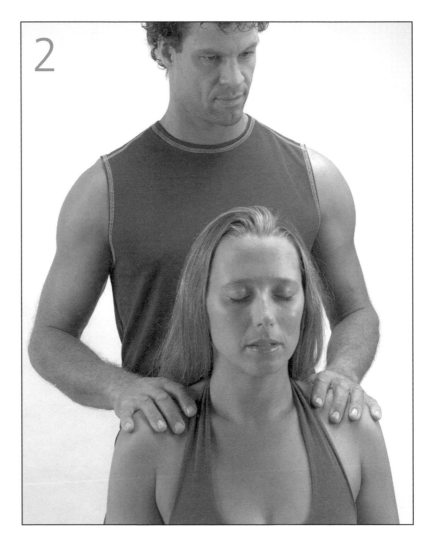

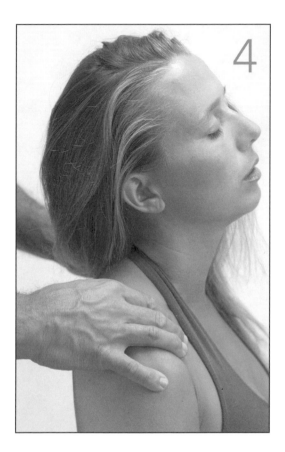

4 Work the muscles from front to back with your fingers and palms, and squeeze them gently in your palms to bring blood to the area. Work together here so the pressure is not too much or too little for the receiver.

5 Watch for the breath. It will tell you a lot. Be patient, since the receiver may want you to work slower or faster or deeper or lighter. Work the shoulders, encouraging release by the kindness of your touch.

6 Begin to move to the neck. Use one hand to support the head at the forehead, as the other works on the neck.

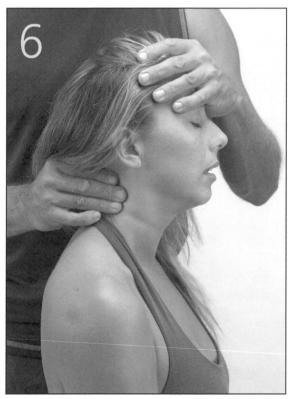

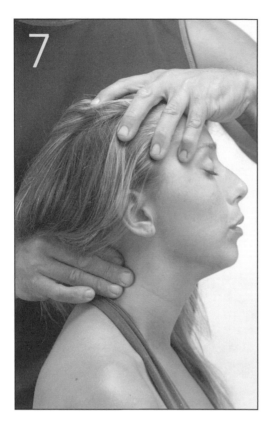

7 Start at the base of the neck and make small circles on either side of the cervical spine, from bottom to top.

8 When you reach the top of the neck, work along the occipital ridge at the hairline, gently pressing the bone where the muscle attaches.

9 Work up into the scalp and use both hands to massage the head and scalp. Work slowly and sensually, and take your time to be gentle and thorough.

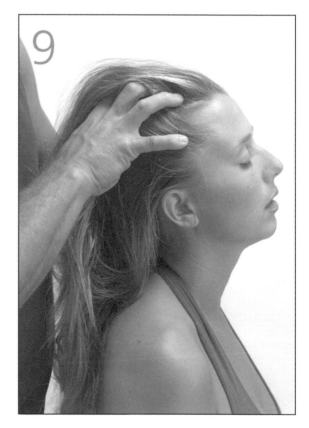

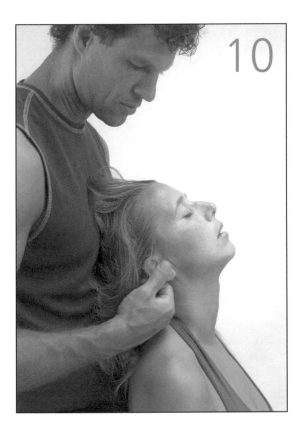

10 Comb your partner's hair with your fingers and gently pull the hair next to the scalp all over the head. If you are standing behind your partner, let her head rest gently on your belly.

11 Take your time and go back and forth from the shoulders to the neck and head, loving your partner in a way that relaxes and nourishes and supports her. A few minutes can go a very long way in making the moment and the evening better for you both. Stroking each other is both natural and instinctive, and you will find wonderful pleasure in discovering creative ways to give and receive touch together.

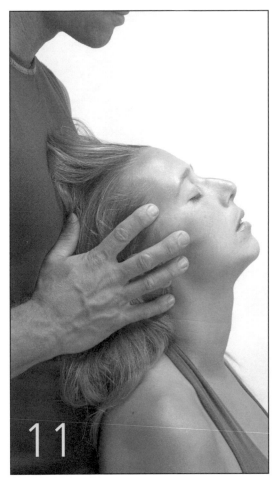

In this chapter, you learned alternative ways of giving each other massage. Spot work or focused work can serve you by addressing specific problem areas and giving the massage a narrower focus. The beautiful backrub, always appreciated, can be given almost anywhere, anytime. You don't even need to remove any clothing. Rather, you can work right through a shirt, as long as loving touch is not limited. Everyone can benefit from this gift, and by offering it freely to each other, you will continue to learn and develop ways to support each other.

CHAPTER 4

THE FOOT MASSAGE

A foot massage has always been a humble expression of love and respect. It is said the ancients and the holy men bestowed it on the most honored and revered. It seems the footbath and massage should have its rightful place within the sharing of lovers, to honor each other in that way also.

For this ritual, you will create some sacred space in which to bathe your lover's feet in herbs and oils, and then to massage them.

PREPARING THE FOOTBATH

You can prepare the herbs in advance by boiling your favorites in water for forty-five minutes, then steeping them for fifteen minutes more. Cool or add cold water. Peppermint is stimulating for the feet; comfrey is good for healing; and rosemary, lavender, and eucalyptus are aromatic and enhance the experience with their rich, sweet smells.

If fresh herbs are not available to you, you can purchase dried ones in any shop that sells herbs. You can also add a few drops of your favorite essential oil to the water as it cools. You can use anything that appeals to you in the moment. Make it sweet or earthy, whatever relaxes you both.

Strain the herb and essential oil mix into a bucket or bowl that is big enough to hold both feet. Don't fill to the top, because it will overflow when the feet go in if it's too full.

Decorate the footbath with flower petals, leaves, and fresh floating flower buds. Cool to a comfortable temperature.

the footbath

1 Choose a quiet space, indoors or out, where you can be together uninterrupted. Place a towel down, put the footbath on top, and place a chair next to it for your partner to sit in while soaking his feet. Make sure the water is cool enough before inviting him to put his feet in the water.

2 As the heat of the water penetrates his grateful feet, allow the aroma of the herbs to bathe you both. After a few moments, gently lift one of your partner's feet in one hand and use your other hand to softly cup the water over it, letting the warm water run over the tops of his feet and between his toes.

3 Hold and caress the foot, and let your touch convey your love for him. Don't be afraid to express it. You are showing honor and respect as well as love by this gesture. Enjoy the humbleness of the act itself. Hold each foot in your hand for a moment, feeling the connection with your partner as you comfort him with your touch.

4 Use a cloth or your hands to wash the feet, gently rubbing the soles, the sides, and the tops of the feet.

5 Touch and lightly massage each foot, as if to give him an appetite for what is to come. Continue this ritual with minimal talk until the water has cooled.

6 Take each foot and dry it carefully and gently, remembering the spaces between and under the toes as well as the heels.

When you have finished, move the herbal bath and bring both feet to rest on the towel. After drying both feet, place your hands on the tops of the feet and hold them there for a moment, as if to assure they are firmly planted on the ground before you move. Slowly break your contact, get up, and stretch your back before going on. Ask your partner to close his eyes and wait for the foot massage to follow.

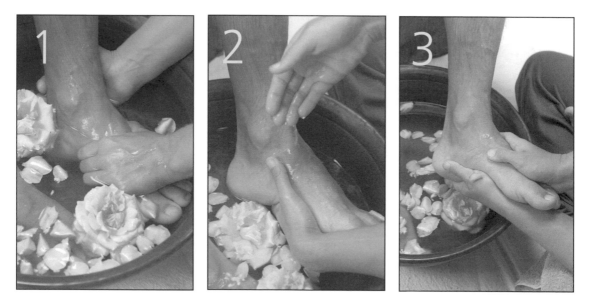

the foot massage

Ideally, you have created a situation where you don't have to move far to be in a comfortable position to give and receive a foot massage. The receiver can be seated comfortably on a chair with her feet in the giver's lap. Another way is to sit on a pillow on the floor, your partner lying faceup. The giver can position himself comfortably, using pillows for support if needed. You can also use the bed, the giver sitting on a chair or stool at the foot of the bed. Sitting at either end of the sofa is a great way to exchange foot massages at the same time.

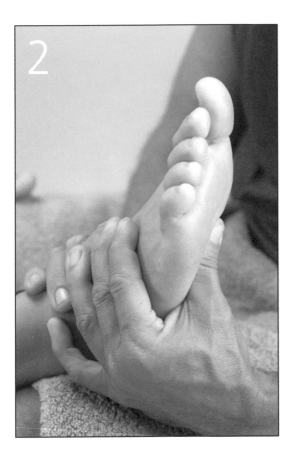

1 Place a soft towel under your partner's feet to protect your lap from the lotion or oil and to make her more comfortable. Take your position on your chair or stool or with her feet on your lap. Sit quietly for a moment. Give yourself the time to be still and relax yourself before beginning to touch your lover's feet.

2 When you are ready, take her feet in your hands and just hold them. Simply be present with your loved one's feet between your palms. Nurture and be nurtured by this sharing.

3 Now, begin to move very slowly and rhythmically, leaning your weight in and out as you hold your partner's feet. Change the positions of your hands, shifting your hold, and continue to move in this way, exploring the movement in the feet.

4 Then oil your hands, and with a firm touch, begin to oil the feet, tops, sides, soles, and toes, and even the valleys between the toes.

5 Once you have oiled the feet well, begin to massage them with love, gently rubbing the soles, the sides, and the tops of the feet in a rhythmic way, so as to help lull your partner into relaxation. Put more lotion on your hands as needed and add some pressure as you work around the heels.

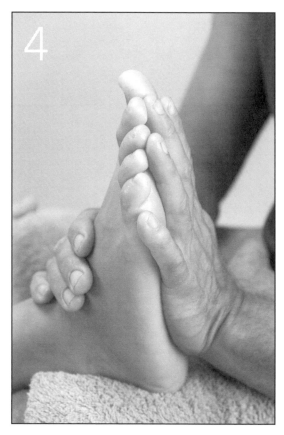

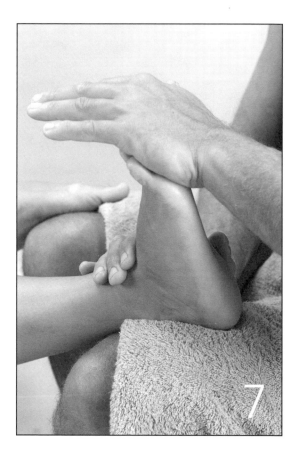

6 Reach up, taking the Achilles tendon between your thumb and finger, and pull and gently squeeze it on your way to the heel.

7 Massage the tops, sides, and soles of the feet.

8 Work the bones back and forth between your palms. Explore the movement of the foot.

9 Use your palms as well as your fingers and thumbs to massage the soles of the feet, and apply enough pressure so your partner is satisfied. Repeat your strokes, and don't be in a rush. Repetition can be mesmerizing and seductive and help your partner sink deeper into relaxation.

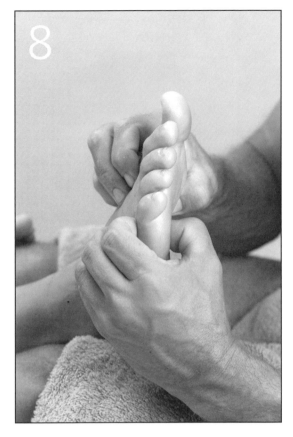

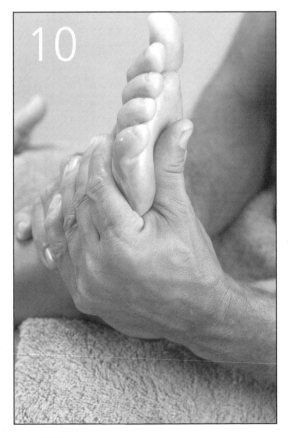

10 Take each toe in your fingers and massage it. Gently lean back to give the joints some traction. Close your eyes. Enjoy simply loving your partner's feet, and express this feeling through your warm and sensitive touch.

completing the foot massage

Work one foot at a time, repeating all the same work on the other foot. Then work them together. Slide your fingers through the spaces between the toes, then flex the foot and rotate the ankle. Rotate one way and then the other. Work as you feel moved and for as long as is comfortable.

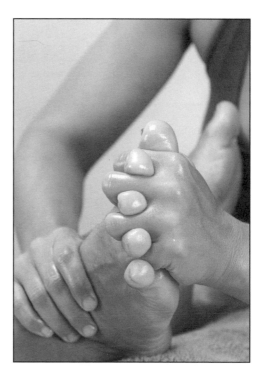

USING A MASSAGE STONE

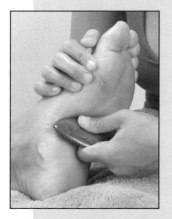

An interesting way to complete your work is to use a tool, a massage stone, such as a piece of jade. Warm it first in the sun or in hot water, as it will pull the body heat from the feet. Find a smooth stone with narrow edges to get in between tendons and toes. Working with the stone can be a very sensual experience for both the giver and the receiver. It will take more awareness and feedback, so that you don't work with too much pressure. It should be soft and sensual. The contrast between the hard stone and your soft, warm hands makes the session that much more interesting. The stone can be used on other parts of the body as well. If an area needs cooling, the cool stone feels great. It can also be heated to warm a tight or cool area of the body.

Watch your lover relax and his breath deepen and tension dissolve as you give this precious gift of a foot massage. Stroke the tops of the feet lightly to end, or find your own way to come to closure. Then simply end as you began, holding your partner's feet warmly in your hands. Stay there for a while before beginning to disconnect. Wipe your lover's feet of any excess lotion or oil, wrap them in a towel, and gently return them to rest. Slowly break your contact, and without words, step away and allow your partner to integrate the work. Encourage him to take her time to experience the wonderful effects of the massage. Wash your hands, and when you're both ready, come together for feedback and exchange.

CHAPTER 5

BUILDING CONNECTION
THROUGH TRUST

This final section of the book offers couples two exercises in trust and awareness. Both of these exercises are wonderful ways to build and develop these qualities, which are so important in a relationship. They can also help in the development of your massage by enhancing your sensitivity and your ability to be present. And mostly they are about taking the time to be with each other, to listen to each other, to support each other, and to rejoice with each other in life's simple and sensual pleasures.

the blind walk exercise

The best place to do this is in nature, where smells, textures, and sounds offer interesting variety. When the ground is uneven, there is an additional element of trust building. However, if it is not possible to do the blind walk outside, you can also explore the indoor space, looking for different tactile sensations, tastes, and smells in your own house. It is good to do this exercise barefoot if the terrain allows.

This will be an exchange. You will need a piece of silk to cover your eyes. If you like, bring along your partner's favorite food. Choose something ripe and sensual, like a mango or a juicy peach, or something rich, like chocolate. Instructions are for the giver unless otherwise noted.

1 Tie the cloth snugly over the receiver's eyes. The first thing the receiver may notice is how his other senses are heightened to compensate for his temporary loss of sight. He cannot move around safely and must depend on you to guide him. Notice any resistance he may have. He may also be delighted and surprised by the experience.

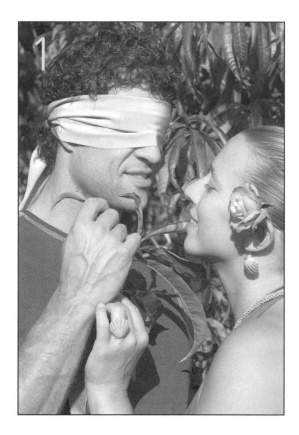

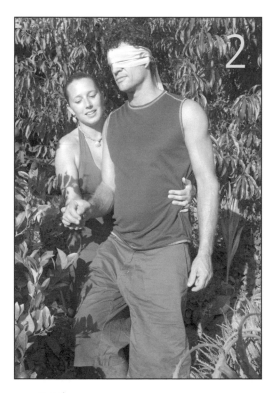

2 With one arm gently around your partner's waist and one supporting his arm, stand together until you both feel grounded and balanced. Make sure the blindfolded partner is comfortable and ready before beginning this adventure into the tactile world.

3 Begin to walk your partner cautiously, giving him plenty of time to move slowly and adjust to this new reality. Walk together for a while to get used to guiding and being guided. Let your partner know in advance about changes in the terrain. Remember, you are his eyes. Move slowly, and notice if your partner can keep up with you or feels rushed. Take your time.

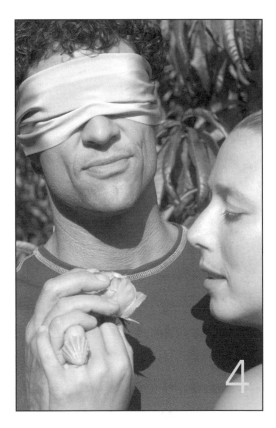

4 When you come to a flower, leaf, a tree, or anything that is interesting, gently stop your partner and lift his hand to touch it. Let him explore the object, identifying it only through touch, smell, or taste. Guide him through a series of tactile, sensual adventures that only your imagination can limit. The receiver will probably begin to realize right away how much he depends on his eyes to identify things, when his other senses are also capable of "seeing." Limit your conversation to what is essential in the moment.

5 Move on and find sweet smells, soft grass, smooth rocks, water, the sound of bells, or the smell of roses. Gently lower your partner to the grass so he can enjoy its softness against his skin. If there is any flat space, roll him on the grass. Let him crawl in the grass.

6 Help him back to his feet. Continue on, then find a place to stop again and sit down, possibly a bench or on the ground or a rock.

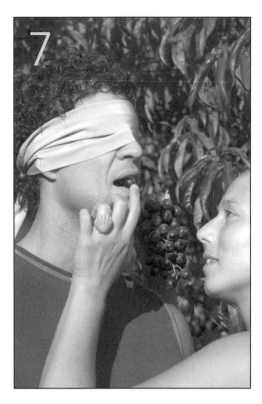

7 If you brought your partner's favorite food, let him hold it and identify it through touch and smell. Then slowly feed it to him. Explore the sensual pleasure of feeding your partner.

8 Wipe his hands and mouth, and continue your walk and exploration. Let your support be firm yet gentle, and find your way back to where you began.

9 Remove the blindfold and take a few minutes to share your experience.

10 Then trade roles and repeat the blind walk, finding a new route.

Let your guidance be gentle and hold each other lightly, giving plenty of space for exploration and trust building. Think about what would bring your partner the most joy in this exercise and do exactly that. Find her favorite flower, fabric, food. Bring her fingers to your own face and let her explore your features with her fingertips. Dip a finger in warm chocolate sauce and let her lick it off.

By exploring the world through touch instead of your eyes, you can greatly expand your sensitivity. You learn to approach things softly on first contact, a good metaphor for life. With each other's loving guidance and support, you can develop trust between you in a very real way through this exploration. The exercise is always new and always fun, so repeat it freely and often, and watch the bonds that you create between you grow.

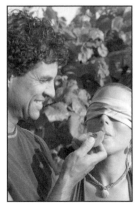

unfolding exercise

Gently unfolding each other from the fetal position to an open, relaxed supine position is an exploration in listening, trust, and letting go. This exercise was developed at Esalen (as was the blind walk) in the early days, when there was a lot of attention given to the teachings of Charlotte Selver. Her sensitivity and awareness trainings were important at a time when people were awakening their sense of bodymind. She taught people how to be still, to listen, to feel, to know themselves inside as well as outside. I learned this exercise from my colleague Vicki Topp, an Esalen teacher and practitioner and cofounder of the Esalen massage school.

Find a comfortable place on the floor or put a mat down to do this exercise. Make sure the room is quiet, warm, and private so you both can focus. Begin with the receiver in the fetal position, with eyes closed, on the mat or rug. The giver prepares, meeting your partner on the floor, kneeling close by but not touching yet. Take a minute to connect to your breath and to center yourself.

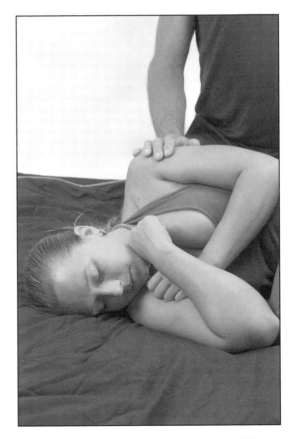

Your exploration will include bringing your partner from the fetal position to the supine, slowly and mindfully, exploring the movement of her body, as if for the first time. You are literally unfolding each other. Listen to your partner's rhythm and let her body speak to you about the pace of your movement. You will begin with the extremities and move to the torso, supporting and opening each joint of the body one by one.

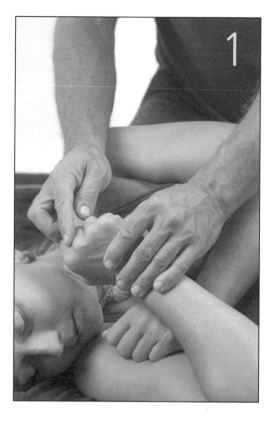

1 Begin with the fingertips of the hand furthest from you. Gently hold your partner's contracted hand in yours, taking time to connect before you begin unfolding.

2 Start by opening each finger, joint by joint, until her palm is facing you.

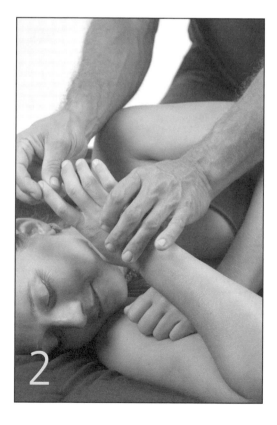

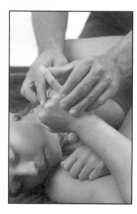

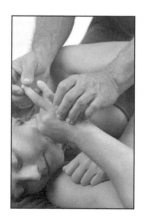

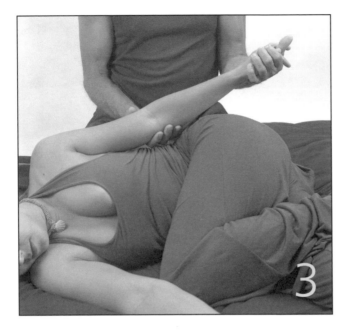

3 Supporting the elbow, slowly open the arm and bring it above the head.

4 Open the other hand in the same way.

5 Now move to the foot of the top leg. Support the knee and foot, and carefully straighten the leg. This will bring the hips over, and you can support the body as it easily rolls to the back.

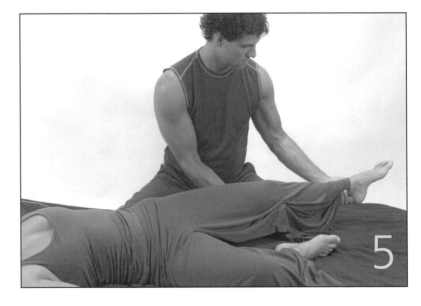

6 Now straighten the other leg, supporting the knee joint as you gently put it down.

7 Make any adjustments to your partner's position to straighten her out. The arms are resting palms up a few inches from her body, and the legs are turned slightly outwards so the feet point away.

8 Come to the head, lift your partner's head, and give a little traction to the neck. Hold her head in your hands, feeling still and connected. Take your time before breaking contact by gently putting her head down on the floor. Slowly come away.

9 Move to the feet, and bending your knees and using your legs to support the weight of your partner's legs, gently lift and rock them back and forth, and then place them back on the floor.

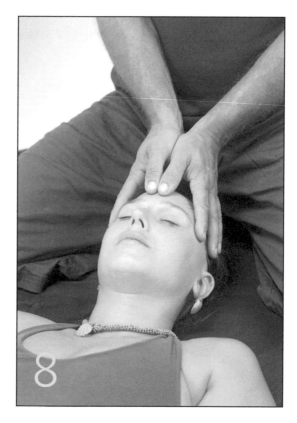

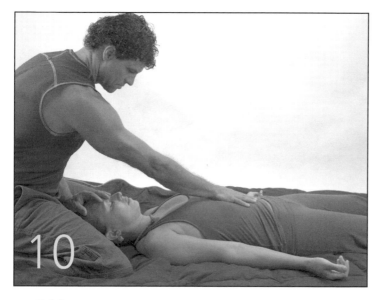

10 Once you have unfolded and opened your partner's body, kneel to one side. Connect with your partner by placing one hand on the belly and the other on the crown of her head. Be still and breathe. Take a moment to be here together before breaking contact.

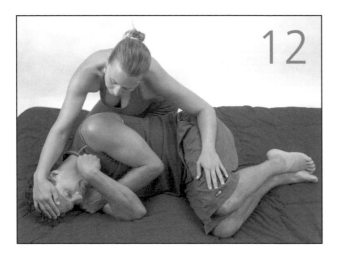

11 Let the receiver return slowly, rolling to the side and pushing up.

12 Change places when you both feel ready. Repeat the exercise.

Exchange feedback after you both have had a turn to give and receive in this exercise. Let your feedback include issues of trust. How did you feel in this practice? Appreciate each other for the time, the attention, and the support. Sometimes feedback is not even necessary as you express feelings of love and compassion by just holding each other.

This exercise will highlight for the receiver the challenge of being completely accepting and letting your lover move you. Release the temptation to help or to control. Imagine that your limbs are sandbags. Accept this passive role for the moment, and let yourself be nurtured and supported. Trust your partner to take loving care of you.

CHAPTER 6

CONCLUSION

By engaging in the art of massage together, you are adding an invaluable practice to your lives, to yourselves, and to your relationship. There are many ways to do massage, and as long as you have your hands and a willingness to give, you need no other tools. The key principles examined in this book in relation to massage are also valuable tools for relationship building. They can be applied to many other areas of your lives as well. Let's review these and see how they apply.

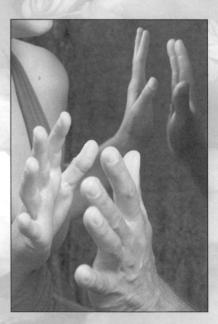

Be centered and present. By

developing your own skills in grounding and centering yourself, you will be better able to deal with all of life's challenges. You have seen the importance of this concept throughout the book, as I have reminded you to ground and center yourself before beginning each massage. You can undoubtedly see other ways to apply this in your own life. Any activity or exchange with each other is more successful if you are both grounded and centered. Then you can be present and you can connect. To make decisions or engage in any kind of deep exchange with each other, it's always better to come from a centered place.

Connection can only happen when both of you are there. Connection is what you long for, not only in massage but in all areas of your lives together. You can use the tools of meditation and awareness to begin to know your breath and to let it take you inside, where there is a refuge and where self-knowledge is always waiting for you. You can learn to connect to yourself and therefore each other. You will learn to trust yourself when acting from this centered place, whatever the circumstances.

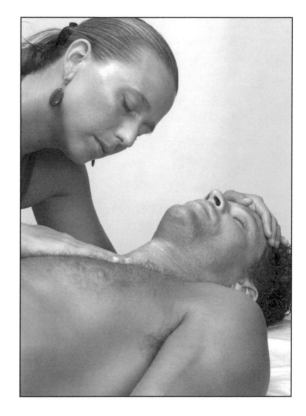

Breathe. Grounding always involves the awareness of breath. Many ancient teachings—such as yoga, tai chi, and the martial arts—teach ways to ground yourself in the physical world and be present in the moment and awake to all that surrounds you. Each of these disciplines has been practiced for thousands of years as a spiritual path, a way to learn about the self and your connection to the whole. All of these practices use breath to begin the journey. As you practice massage and start to pay attention to your breathing, this awareness will carry over to other situations where remembering just to breathe is the best choice of action in the moment.

Approach each other with tenderness and respect.

Let your initial touch be slow and easy as you enter each other's space with awareness. The same can apply to your everyday contact with each other. Develop your awareness and sense of timing, so you approach each other gently, without invading each other's space. In order to be heard, you must see. Let your timing include awareness and consideration of each other. For example, if your partner has just returned home from work, see her need for time to transition. Wait a little while before seeking her full attention. Feel each other's space before you enter it. Your love is manifest in your consideration of each other.

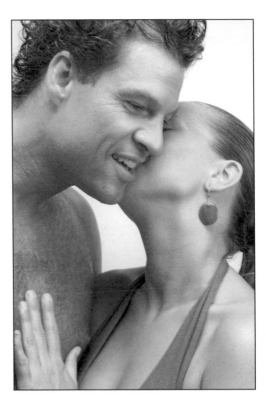

Listen to each other. Communicate your needs.

Learning to listen to each other and to hear what your partner is asking for will go a long way in improving the quality of your contact. As you begin to massage each other and practice communicating specifically about what you need, this can carry over to other aspects of the relationship, such as lovemaking, and what you want for your birthday, and all kinds of things. In a marriage, you can't read each other's minds, and most people need to tell their partner what they want. To expect anyone to read your mind will not get you what you want. You must ask, and in massage, you must ask and also give feedback. Positive feedback goes miles in making each other feel good. You will learn to quickly respond to feedback in massage and to not take the information your partner gives you personally or as a criticism. Work on making your feedback to each other balanced, with positive feedback as well as suggestions for improvement. Learn to be specific about your needs. This means you must be honest with yourself and with each other. Learning to communicate lovingly and honestly is a skill that can be learned and developed. There are classes and workshops offered for couples worldwide in developing these skills.

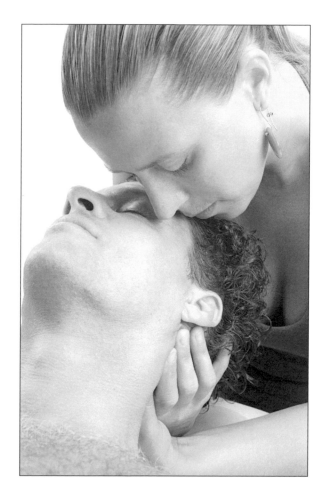

One of the objectives in massage is to support your partner, both physically and emotionally. You are supporting each other's need to relax, to heal, and to be nurtured and to be touched. By attending to each other's pain, you are developing your compassion for each other and deepening your love by your willingness to be there for each other. Working together will reinforce this support for you both. It will also help you to develop the trust and the security that provide a solid foundation for the relationship to deepen and grow. Let your feelings of tenderness express themselves through your touch.

Use this book as a guide to developing your touch as well as an introduction to gentle massage techniques. Try the full body massage exchange, the spot work, and the explorations into trust and sensation. Find ways to touch each other and make some time to be together. Life can be demanding, and you're pulled in many directions. Remember to nourish your relationship. Develop a practice of being together in a meaningful way. By making a commitment to this, you are affirming your commitment to each other and to making change in your relationship in a positive way. Stay connected by sharing your loving touch. Let the gift of giving massage to each other manifest its goodness in your lives.

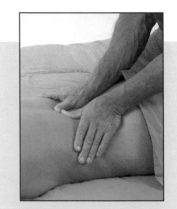

LEARN MASSAGE AT ESALEN

If you become enchanted with massage, as happened for me, I highly recommend a course at Esalen Institute, renowned for its holistic approach and excellence in massage and bodywork. Courses in massage are presented regularly.

PEGGY MORRISON HORAN is a thirty-five-year practitioner and teacher of Esalen Massage, student of yoga and movement, and retired midwife. She coproduced the Esalen Massage Video in 1996 and was one of the founders of the Esalen Massage School. She managed the Massage Department at Esalen for many years before retiring from management in 2004. She still practices and teaches there.

Foreword writer GABRIELLE ROTH is the creator of the Five-Rhythms Movement Meditation Practice. She is a theater director and the author of *Maps to Ecstacy: The Healing Power of Movement.*

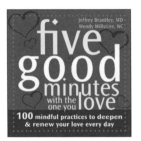
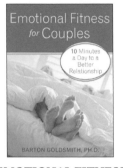
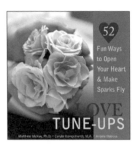
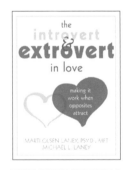
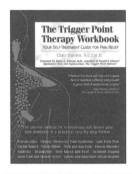
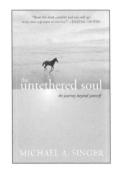
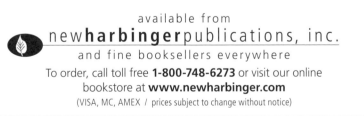